SPORT TOURISM

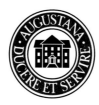

SPORT TOURISM

Douglas Michele Turco

Illinois State University

Roger Riley

Winona State University

Kamilla Swart

Account Director, Octagon South Africa

Fitness Information Technology, Inc.

•

P.O. Box 4425

•

Morgantown, WV 26504-4425

Library of Congress Card Catalog Number: 02-102223

ISBN: 1-88-5693-43-5

Copyeditor: Sandra Woods
Cover Design: Krazy Kat Designs
Managing Editor: Geoffrey C. Fuller
Developmental Editor: Jessica E. McDonald
Production Editor: Craig Hines
Proofreader: Maria denBoer
Indexer: Maria denBoer
Printer: Data Reproductions

10   9   8   7   6   5   4   3   2   1

Fitness Information Technology, Inc.
P.O. Box 4425, University Avenue
Morgantown, WV 26504 USA
800.477.4348
304.599.3483 phone
304.599.3482 fax
Email: fit@fitinfotech.com
Website: www.fitinfotech.com

Contents

Preface xv
Introduction xvii

CHAPTER 1

Defining Sport Tourism 1

CHAPTER 2

The Sport Tourism Industry 23

CHAPTER 3

Making Dollars and Sense:
Economic Impacts of Sport Tourism 53

CHAPTER 4

Defining Sport Tourism Events 73

CHAPTER 5

Conducting Sport Tourism Events:
Strategies for Implementation 111

CHAPTER 6

Evaluating Sport Tourism 147

CHAPTER 7

Financing Sport Tourism 163

CHAPTER 8

Professional Preparation in Sport Tourism 183

CHAPTER 9

Issues in Sport Tourism 213

CHAPTER 10

Future Directions in Sport Tourism 225

References 255
Index 265
About the Authors 279

Photo Credits

Detailed Contents

Chapter 1: Defining Sport Tourism

What Is Sport Tourism. 3

Models of Sport Tourism 4

Intensity of Involvement in Sport Tourism. 10

Sport—Guiding Descriptions 14

What Is Tourism?. 17

Chapter 2: The Sport Tourism Industry

Introduction 23

The Sport Industry 23

The Sport Tourism System. 24

Problems of Providing Sport Tourism Services 41

The Sport Tourist—Behavior and Motivations. 44

Sport Tourism as a Distinct Market Niche 48

Unique Characteristics of the Sport Tourism Markets 51

Chapter 3: Making Dollars and Sense: Economic Impacts of Sport Tourism

Introduction 53

Economic Impact. 53

Economic Costs in Sport 58

Econometric Models 65

Issues in Economic Impact Research 66

Discussion Questions. 72

Chapter 4: Designing Sport Tourism Events

Introduction 73

Definition of Sport Tourism Events 74

Importance of Research 74

Informal Assessment of the Need to Host an Event 74

Formal Appraisal of the Need to Host an Event 75

Feasibility Study. 76

A "Yes" Feasibility Study 81

Event Bidding Considerations 81
Sport Tour: Five Still Alive as IOC Makes Cruelest Cut 83
Planning Considerations 85
Market Planning Considerations 86
Market Segments 88
Values Attitudes and Lifestyles (VALS) 90
Sport Tourist Destination Area (STDA) Characteristics 92
Business Planning Considerations 94
Strategic Planning Considerations 95
Organizational Structure 101
Setting and Location Considerations 104
Free Versus Paid Admission 107
Factors Related to Poor Events 107
Future Considerations 108
Summary 109
Discussion Questions 110

**Chapter 5: Conducting Sport Tourism Events:
Strategies for Implementation**
Introduction 111
Administrative Strategies 112
Sport Tour: Volunteer Services Subcommittee for the
    8th World Swimming Championships, Perth, 1998 116
Community Involvement Strategies 124
Quality Service Strategies 124
Operations Plan 125
Sponsorship Strategies 139
Wrap-Up and Evaluation Strategies 143
Summary 144
Discussion Assignments 145

Chapter 6: Evaluating Sport Tourism
Introduction 147
Sport Tourist Satisfaction 148
Sponsorship Evaluation 148
Issues in Sport Tourism Evaluation 150
Sampling 153
Survey Location and Scheduling 155
Determining Sport Tourist Groups 156
Sport Tourism Research: Longitudinal Approaches 157
Residents' Perceptions of Sport Tourism 158
Summary 161

Chapter 7: Financing Sport Tourism

Introduction 163
Sport Tourism Revenue Sources 163
Earned Income. 165
Sport Tourism Pricing Policies 166
Sponsorship Decision-Making 168
Sponsorship Benefits 169
Sponsorship Considerations 174
Sport Sponsorship Issues 175
Tobacco Sponsorship in Sport 176
Financing Sport Tourism Capital Development 178
Grants 181
Summary 182
Sponsorship Resources 182

Chapter 8: Professional Preparation in Sport Tourism

Introduction 183
Websites for Sports Managment/Tourism/Recreation Programs:
    Undergraduate and Graduate 185
Core Content of Graduate Studies 186
Service Learning: Internships, Practicums,
    and Fieldwork Experiences 188
Websites for Internships and Jobs. 192
Seeking Employment 196
Professional Associations 200
Networking 201
Evaluating Your Current and Future Network 202
Professional Organizations 204
Additional Resources 206
Major League Baseball Franchises. 209
NBA Franchises 210
NFL Franchises 211
NHL Franchises. 212

Chapter 9: Issues in Sport Tourism

Introduction 213
Urban Sport-Facility Development 214
Sport Gambling. 218
Atlantic City, New Jersey vs. Las Vegas, Nevada 219
Racing 220
Overcommercialization of Sport. 221
Discussion Questions—Sport Commercialization 222

Chapter 10: Future Directions in Sport Tourism

Trends vs. Fads. 226
General Tourism Trends. 228
Demographics 232
Motivations, Lifestyles, and Sports Tourism Futures. 236
Extreme Sports. 238
Technology and Sport Tourism Futures 241
The Rise of the NASCAR Fan Base 248
The Economic Power of Sport Tourism 250
Sport Tourism Marketplace 250

Text Graphics List

Chapter 1 • 1

Summary Questions. 1
Some Facts and Figures 2
Figure 1.1 The Sport Tourism Phenomenon Model 4
Cruises for the Avid Golfer 5
Golf Tourism 6
Disney Sports Resort 6
Sport and Tourism 8
Figure 1.3 The Getty Model. 9
Figure 1.4 Demand Side Sports Behavior. 11
Figure 1.5 Supply Side Sports Behavior 13
What is Your Definition of Sport 16
Figure 1.6 Top 10 World Destinations 18
Figure 1.7 U.S. Domestic Tourism. 19
Figure 1.8 U.S. International Tourism 20

Chapter 2 • 23

Summary Questions. 23
Fluctuations in the Tourism Market. 25
Figure 2.1 The sport tourism system 26
Figure 2.2 Internet Usage by American Travelers—2000 29
Figure 2.3 Transportation Methods of U.S. Travelers—2000 30
Table 2.1 The Largest U.S. and International
    Common Carrier Airlines—2000 31
Table 2.2 Twenty Busiest Airports in the World 2000 34
Table 2.3 Secondary Tourist Attractions. 37
Political Turmoil in New Zealand Sport Tourism 40
Table 2.4 Personality Types and Travel Propensities 47
Sport Tour: Cape Town, South Africa 50
Sport Tour: New Zealand. 51
Sport Tour: Green Bay, Wisconsin 52

Chapter 3 • 53

Summary Questions. 53
Figure 3.1 55
Demonstrating Value of Event or Operations. 55
Assisting in Attracting Sponsorships. 56
Generating Consumer Market Profile 57
Helping to Gain Public Sector Support
    for Sport Tourism Operations 57
Sources of Economic Impact at Sport Tourism Events 60
Local economy. 60
Table 3.1 Examples of Designated Economies
    of Impact in Sport Tourism 61
Figure 3.2 Essential Economic Impact Survey Questions 62
Table 3.2 Table of nonresident spectators. 64
Table 3.4 Direct Economic Impact of
    the National Bicycling Championships 65
Sport Tourism Event Spending Profiles 71
Sport Tour: It Pays to Play 72

Chapter 4 • 73

Summary Questions. 73
Blue Blood Estates 91
New Melting Pot 91
Types of Sport Tourism Resources 92
Sport Tourism Development Action Strategies. 94
Sport Tour: Vodacom Beach Africa 98
Sport Tour: Tour de France Doping Scandal 99
Figure 4.1 A Simple Organizational Structure 101
Figure 4.2 FINA 8th World Swimming
    Championships Organization 102
Figure 4.3 Example of a Sport Tourism
    Organizational Structure 103

Chapter 5 • 111

Summary Questions. 111
Sport Tour: Volunteer Services Coordinator—Duty Statements
    for the 8th World Swimming Championships, Perth 1998 116
Sport Tour: The Hillsborough Disaster 123
Sport Tour: Old Mutual Two Oceans Marathon. 136
Sport Tour: World Cup Travel Services
    for World Cup USA '94 138
Sport Tour: Buffed Bods, Big Crowds Spell Bonanza
    for Beach Volleyball. 140

Chapter 6 • 147

Summary Questions. 147
Table 6.1 Summary of Field Survey Techniques
    Used in Sport Tourism Event Research 151
Sample Size 154
Table 6.2 Sport Tourism Event Sample Sizes
    and Precision Levels. 155
Table 6.3 Survey Schedule—1992 ASA Men's Fast Pitch
    Softball World Championship Tournament. 156
Sport Tour: 13th Asian Games. 157
Sport Tour: Kodak Albuquerque International Balloon Fiesta 160

Chapter 7 • 163

Summary Questions. 163
Table 7.1 Sport Tourism Revenue Classifications and Types. 164
Principle 1: Participants Seek Fairness in Pricing 167
Principle 2: Consumers Seek Value 167
Principle 3: Consumers Seek Choices. 167
Table 7.2 Corporate Benefits of Sport Sponsorship 169
Figure 7.1 171
Sport Tour: NASCAR Is Moving Up 174
Figure 7.2 176
A Comparison of General Obligation and Revenue Bonds. 179

Chapter 8 • 183

Summary Questions. 183
Table 8.1 Content Areas of Academic Programs in Tourism. 188
Organizations Involved in Sport Tourism. 198

Chapter 9 • 213

Summary Questions. 213
Trends and Related Issues. 213
Sport Tour: Traveling With the NFL Rams 216

Chapter 10 • 225

Summary Questions. 225
Figure 10.1 Revent Growth Rate in World Tourism Receipts. 229
Figure 10.2 Projected International
    Tourism Arrivals Until 2020 229
Table 10.1 Top Ten Tourists Destinations—1998. 230
Table 10.2 Top Ten Tourists Destinations—2020. 230
Figure 10.3 World Population Projection Until 2200. 233
Table 10.3 Populations by Regions of the World 234

Table 10.4 Income Per Capita of People in
   Developed and Developing Nations 235
Table 10.5 Average Number of Vacation Days
   of Countries Around the World. 240
Figure 10.4 International Spending on the Internet 244
Table 10.6 Projected Growth of Travel Revenue
   on the Internet (US$billions) 245
Figure 10.5 United States Internet Spending
   Comparisons by Products 245

Preface

Sport and tourism have grown increasingly close during recent years and have developed into a distinct niche market. Consequently, sport tourism is slowly gaining recognition as an academic discipline in its own right, with many institutions worldwide offering sport tourism degrees and courses. The purpose of this text is to provide students with a solid foundation of the sport tourism knowledge and issues that are embedded in the larger industries of tourism and sport provision. Numerous sport tours are included as resources to depict different aspects of the sport tourism industry. Since sport tourism is a global occurrence, these sport tours have been specifically selected to illustrate the effects of sport tourism in different corners of the globe.

Sport Tourism has four distinct sections. The first two chapters provide the reader with a foundation of knowledge related to sport tourism, including definitions of sport and tourism, various models of the sport tourism industry, and an exploration of the workings of the sport and tourism industries. The next five chapters focus on specific aspects of event-based sport tourism, which is given prominence in this text as its attributes are easier to quantify and observe than the attributes of participatory sport tourism. Chapter 3 describes the economic costs and benefits of sport tourism and explains methods to assess the economic impacts of sport tourism. As sport tourism events are globally significant in terms of their ability to generate popular appeal and attract investment, chapters 4 and 5 focus on key considerations for successful sport tourism events and strategies for implementation. Chapter 6 focuses on why sport tourism event organizers evaluate their services and describes various types of evaluations that are timely to managers. Chapter 7 completes this section by describing common methods of financing sport tourism facilities and service operations. The third section of the text examines professional preparation in sport tourism. Chapter 8 discusses academic competencies and service learning and professional associations and provides the student with useful contact details of institutions, organizations, and professional associations involved in the sport tourism industry. The fourth and final section of the text looks at issues in sport tourism today and provides some thought on the future direction of sport tourism. Several issues, such as sport facility financing, sport gambling, and over-commercialization of sport and host-guest interactions, are discussed in Chapter 9. In Chapter 10, we speculate on the future of sport tourism by examining general tourism trends, as well as general and business occurrences that could influence the future of sport tourism.

Overall, this text provides the reader with foundational knowledge of sport tourism. Not only will *Sport Tourism* add to the limited resources focusing exclusively on sport tourism, but it will also invoke inquiring thought among both students and sport tourism professionals and prove a valuable resource to those seeking employment in the field.

Introduction

If you are a teacher, sports program administrator, tourism professional, or a student preparing for a career in sports tourism, this book will introduce you to some of the concepts, practices, and issues that belong to this industry. Sports is the attraction or activity that lures people to places, and tourism combines various means to bring people to different geographical locations to engage in that attraction or activity.

The material used in this book is designed for the novice reader and the interested professional, but mostly it gives the reader an overview of a rapidly growing segment of the tourism industry. Until recently, tourism was indescribable because there were no uniformly gathered statistics and no parameters defining the tourism industry. These problems were removed in recent years, and the sub-segment of sports tourism can now be defined, described, and passed on to you, the reader.

There is some debate over whether the activities in this book should be considered sports, and therefore warrant inclusion under the umbrella of sport tourism. *Sport Tourism* intentionally offers a wide view of the industry so that all readers will be able to find activities that meet their definitions and address their needs. The book takes novice readers through various descriptions of sports tourism and the sports tourism industry before delving into important practices such as designing, implementing and evaluating sports tourism events. The book also contains all-important chapters on the financing of sports tourism and on issues related to economic impacts. In the final chapters, professional preparation and the future of sport tourism are addressed.

How to Use the Book

When reading books, people tend to get bogged down in the text and need a break from the concepts being offered. Our suggestion is that readers review the *Questions* at the start of each chapter so they keep focused on the meanings of the text and its concepts. We also suggest that readers take a break and read the case studies interspersed throughout the text. Not only will the case studies provide a respite from the text, but they will also illustrate abstract concepts with real-life examples. In addition to case studies, several chapters include how-to steps that can be followed when trying to apply the concepts to practical situations. These steps have been used by the authors and their students on several occasions and have always proved successful.

About the Authors

There are several bonds that connect the authors to each other, although they now live in geographically disparate parts of the world. First, we all worked or studied at Illinois State University —although at different times; second, we all have backgrounds in both sports and in tourism research (with varying levels of success in sports but more success in our tourism research); and third, we are all keen travelers of the world. At some point in time, we have collectively visited every continent and collectively engaged, organized, or viewed hundreds of sporting events. With Kamilla in South Africa, and Doug and Roger in the United States, it difficult to say when all the authors will be in the same place again. Such is the way of the global world. But with the Internet, a keystroke or two, and the press of a "Send" button, we can be instantaneously connected.

Chapter 1

Defining Sport Tourism

Questions

1. What is sport tourism?
2. What is the relationship between sport and tourism?
3. What are the benefits of participation in sport tourism?
4. Why is sport tourism a distinct market niche within the broader tourism industry?
5. What significant events or movements have shaped the sport tourism industry?

As can be seen in the statistics on the next page (see *Some Facts and Figures*), tourism is a huge industry. It is equally clear that *sport tourism* is a vital segment of this growing business. This book provides an overview of sport tourism and its place within the larger industries of tourism and sport provision. A number of issues related to sport tourism are explored in the hope that, when they are finished, readers will better understand the potentials and pitfalls.

The reader will also have a variety of resource inserts, "Sport Tours," that will illustrate some aspects of the sport tourism phenomenon. Readers will "travel" to various locales including New Zealand; Green Bay, Wisconsin; and Cape Town, South Africa to further understand the concepts and definitions previously covered.

In this chapter, the reader is provided with a foundation of knowledge related to sport tourism, including definitions of sport, tourism, and sport tourism.

Gibson (1998b) contends that there is an international divide in the field of sport tourism, with two distinct perspectives: *active or participatory sport tourism* and *event-based sport tourism*. The Europeans (De Knopf & Standevan, 1998) tend to define sport tourism in terms of the active participant (e.g., cross-country skiing, playing golf or tennis). Conversely, much of the work in the United States defines sport tourism as event-based spectating, with the sport participants being the athletes. There may be a third form of sport tourism, which centers on sport halls of fame, stadia, cruises, and themed eating and drinking places (Gibson, 1998a; Gibson, Attle, & Yiannakis, 1998), that we term *celebratory sport tourism*. This book aims for a unified field to cover all kinds of sport tourism. We contend that three types of sport tourism must be accommodated in any legitimate discussion of sport tourism as a singular field of study. Most of the examples in this book come from event-based sport tourism because its attributes (marketing, sponsorship, economic impact, etc.) are easier to quantify and observe than are the attributes of participatory sport tourism (wonderful streams for fishing, amazing nature trails, outstanding golf courses). This is not to imply that the other types of sport tourism are not as important. The rise in event-based sport tourism is attributed to the popularity of active sport tourism experiences.

Some Facts and Figures

The Travel Industry Association of America (TIAA) statistics for travel and tourism in 1997 are impressive. In the United States, travel and tourism expenditures amounted to $473 billion. Travel and tourism was one of the largest industries in the country generating 6.6 million jobs directly and $116 billion in payroll. Indirect jobs amounted to another 8.9 million positions. TIAA claimed that once again, tourism was the United States' leading export with 46.3 million visiting tourists spending $90 billion. The positive balance of payments for 1996 [foreigners spending money in the United States versus Americans spending money outside the United States] was a record $26 billion. International visitors spent $247 million every day. Imagine the dollars that were generated and jobs that were created when domestic travel and tourism [Americans traveling within the United States] were factored into the totals. (National Society for Park Resources, 1998).

It is estimated that sport tourism is growing at an annual rate of 8–10% (Delpy, 1997).

The Sport Tourism Study done for the Texas Department of Economic Development (1997) estimated that the events had economic impacts on their communities:

Sporting Event	City in Texas	Economic Impact
1994 Soccer World	Dallas	$301,000,000
1996 Houston Livestock Show and Rodeo	Houston	$150,000,000
1994 Mobil Cotton Bowl (college football)	Dallas	$ 56,500,000
1995 Senior Sports Classic	San Antonio	$ 4,700,000

(based on average spending of $100 per day per visitor)

Smaller sporting events can have substantial economic impacts on their communities. The Irving (Texas) Chamber of Commerce estimated that a high school football play-off game generated more economic activity from accommodations and sales tax than a Dallas Cowboys football game. (Texas Department of Economic Development, 1997).

What Is Sport Tourism?

General Description

Sport tourism includes travel to and participation in or attendance at a predetermined sport activity. The sport activity can include competition and travel for recreation, entertainment, business, education and/or socializing. The sport can be competitive and/or recreational. (Texas Department of Economic Development, 1997).

An Overview of Sport-Tourism Relationships

Sport has been defined in many ways. It typically refers to physically oriented activity guided by an organized format and rules that are imposed by participants or an organized body that represents the sport. The goals of the sport are usually to beat an opponent, compete against a standard of performance, or achieve a predetermined goal. However, a broader definition of sport is required when addressing sport tourism. According to this definition, sport is any activity, experience, or production for which the primary focus is athletics or physical recreation. For example, a person who enjoys fishing may enter a contest to catch the largest fish under rules of time and specific areas to fish. According to the first definition, these people are engaged in a sport by virtue of the rules and the competition. However, according to the second rendition of sport, people are no less involved in sport if they decide to drive 100 miles to engage in fishing for the enjoyment of catching and releasing fish.

Attractions are the primary lure for destinations that entice visitors, and sport is an important attraction for many people. Other tourism attractions may be categorized within the contexts of cultural, historic, environmental, or social realms. Sport tourism can also serve as a supplemental, secondary, or peripheral attraction within host communities. That is, the primary reason for visiting a destination is not sports but other types of attractions. While visiting a destination, tourists visit a sports attraction to supplement their activities or to fill time between other planned activities. Sport, as a supplemental or secondary attraction, can be used to further satisfy visitors' needs, extend their length of stay in the host community, and stimulate economic activity. In many cases, conference and convention sites are purposely selected by virtue of their sporting facilities, such as golf and tennis centers, and recognized sports events (secondary attraction) that will entertain visiting delegates after their business is complete. Hallmark sporting events such as the Olympics can attract many tourists even when they have little knowledge of or interest in a sport. These sporting events are of worldwide, regional or national importance in terms of their visibility, and they typically foster other attractions that seek to capitalize on the increased tourist volume. Although one person visits the primary sporting attraction, their companions may visit the other attractions.

Sport tourists are those people who visit a destination for the primary purpose of participating in or viewing sport. There are a myriad of sport tourism examples, from the traditional resorts that attract skiers, golfers, and tennis players to the more extreme sport opportunities, such as rock-climbing locations. Sport tourists can attend a World Cup match in Great Britain or compete in a youth hockey tournament in Quebec. Sport tourism can also include fantasy camps where adults spend a week or more with former athletes by training and competing in a particular sport or attendance at sport-related museums (Turco & Eisenhart, 1998).

Models of Sport Tourism

Several sport tourism models have been used to explain the phenomenon. Although any model can be criticized as not being complete, the depiction of models allows for discussion and understanding of the phenomenon from different perspectives. The models discussed in the following section include (a) the sports tourism phenomenon model (Kurtzman & Zauhar, 1997), (b) the sports tourism definition model (Gammon & Robinson, 1997), (c) the sport-event model of supply and demand (Getz, 1998), and our (d) intensity of involvement in sport tourism model.

The first of these models (Kurtzman & Zauhar, 1997) is designed to integrate sport tourism motivation with destinations and settings that serve sport tourists. The model also suggests other types of tourism that may contribute to the sport tourism phenomenon in particular circumstances.

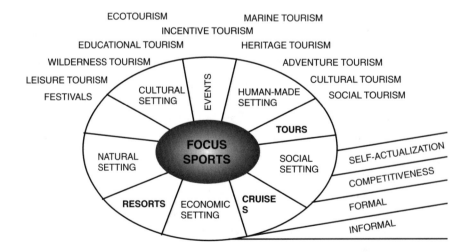

Figure 1.1. The Sports Tourism Phenomenon Model

The darkened area called "Focus Sports" denotes the hub of this model. With the focus of sport tourism being sporting activities (competitive or recreational, participant, official or spectator), it is the core from which the phenomenon is generated.

Denoted by the words in bold type, the spokes are the types of tourism modalities that involve sport tourism. In this respect, sport tourism takes place at, within, or on cruise ships, tours, resorts, other attractions, and special events. Each sport tourism setting will be described in the following sections.

- *Cruises.* Oftentimes cruise lines will organize specialty cruises where sports celebrities are invited to join the passengers for a particular sporting theme. Some of these cruises focus on golf with instruction on board and golf games at every port of call. However, a sport cruise also could be a Chicago Cubs baseball cruise where members of the professional baseball team join the passengers to relive the past season in conversations and discussions. Alternatively, a sport cruise could be oriented to engaging in, learning about, or competing in a variety of other sporting activities.

- *Tours.* Sport tours can involve many varieties of observing or playing sport. A tour may involve a bus trip that takes sport tourists to 10 baseball games in 10 different stadiums during a 15-day span. A sport tour could also include a package of Rugby World Cup games in the United Kingdom with accommodations, transportation, food, and other types of entertainment. Sport tours may also be organized by individual tourists using already existing attractions and services. Such a case is the state of Alabama, which heavily promotes its Robert Trent Jones Golf Trail. This trail touts several golf courses by the famous course designer that are open to the public. Avid golfers are encouraged to take their own car to all these courses or to call and have arrangements made for them.

- *Resorts.* Sport resorts are those resorts where tourists learn, practice and play their chosen sport. Although accommodations and other services are provided on site, the primary focus is the sport. Alternatively, many resorts offer fantasy camps where sport enthusiasts can experience the activities of professional sports training camp with retired veterans of the game. Some resorts specialize in one sport whereas others try to encompass a wider share of the market by offering many sports for either viewing or participation. In the case of the new Disney World sport complex, the variety of sports packages is astounding.

- *Other attractions.* Sporting attractions can involve anything that lures tourists because a particular sport is emphasized. From a sports hall of fame (e.g., Cooperstown, New York, baseball; Canton, Ohio, football) to sporting museums, to sports-themed restaurants and bars, a sporting attraction need not encompass competitive event. The "Field of Dreams" baseball diamond in Dyersville, Iowa, can easily be a sports attraction as can sports facilities and sports conventions or products shows. Tours of Wimbledon, the Indianapolis Motor Speedway, and the manufacturing plant of the Louisville Slugger baseball bat attract thousands of visitors annually. One could make the case that tours of the Roman Coliseum would also fall in this category of sport tourism attractions.

- *Events.* Sporting events are contests and activities that sport tourists visit to participate in, organize, officiate at, or observe. These are the most common types of sporting activities for sports tourists. In addition, sporting events can be the celebration or commiseration of an event won or lost. After each of the Chicago Bulls victories in the

Golf Tourism

According to Tom Nutley of Reed Travel Exhibitions, golf-related travel is one of the fastest growing segments of the tourism industry. The International Association of Golf Tours Operators estimated the global value of golf tourism to exceed $5 billion per year. The CEO of Brice International, a New York-based golf tour operator estimates the average golf trip has four people, and they each pay about $2,500 to $3,000, not including airfares. The National Golf Foundation's 1995 research report said there were 10.5 million golf tourists playing 62 million rounds and representing 14% of all golf in the United States each year. During 1994, nearly half of the adult golfing population took at least one golf-related trip.

Source: *"Advertisement for Themed,"* 1998.

Disney Sports Resort

The Walt Disney Co. in Orlando, Florida, has developed spectator and participant sports activities into its packages to attract a new niche market. In early 1998, there were events such as the Walt Disney World Marathon, World Series of Baseball Fantasy Camp, Chevy Trucks Motor Racing, Indy 200 Stock Car Race, Atlanta Braves Spring Training (baseball), Bryant Gumbel-Walt Disney World Golf Tournament, and the Amateur Athletic Union Karate World Championships. If sports tourists stay for 3 nights or more, they can pay an additional $32 for golf, tennis, water craft rental, water skiing, horseback riding, fishing, and health club admission. For an additional fee, rock climbing is available at the Disney Institute and scuba diving at the Living Seas Pavilion in the Epcot Center. Snorkeling is also available at the Shark Reef of Typhoon Lagoon.

Source: *"Disney Complex,"* 1997.

NBA Championship game, people from all over the country gathered in Grant Park, on the Chicago waterfront, to see and hear their champions in person.

The spoke interspaces. For Kurtzman and Zauhar (1997), the spoke interspaces are the types of environments where sports tourism can occur:

- Human-Made Settings—stadiums, museums, cruise boats

- Social Settings—bars, restaurants, cities

- Economic Settings—trade shows and conventions

- Natural Settings—mountains, lakes, beaches, rivers, in the air

- Cultural Settings—rodeos in Texas, bullfights in Spain

The outer rim. The outer rim of this sport tourism model refers to other types of tourism where sport tourism can also occur. For example, in the types of tourism that use the natural resources as their attraction (ecotourism, wilderness tourism, marine tourism, and typically adventure tourism), many sports are conducted either competitively or recreationally. Scuba diving, cross-country skiing, fishing, mountaineering, and whitewater kayaking are a few of the most apparent sports. In types of tourism that fit into social or cultural realms (heritage tourism, cultural tourism, social tourism), sports may be part of the social or cultural attractions within that location. Elephant soccer in Asia, any soccer in Brazil, or "Golden Oldies" tournaments all make up part of the social and cultural fabric of particular destinations.

The roadway. To the right-hand side of the Kurtzman and Zauhar (1997) model are the various motivations that may drive a person to engage in sport tourism. These motivations are set in a tiered form (a wavy road for Kurtzman & Zauhar) to denote that sport tourists can move from one form of motivation to another depending on their needs, wants, or desires. These types of motivations are

- Informal sports—to participate or spectate for recreational purposes

- Formalized sports—to participate or spectate at organized sporting events

- Competitive sports—to participate or spectate at competitions

- Self-Actualization—to participate or spectate for intrinsic benefits

The Sport Tourism Definition Model

The sport tourism model of Gammon and Robinson (1997) classifies various types of sport tourist activities. The classification system describes sport tourists by the activities they undertake while traveling and by their primary or secondary motivation to engage in sports while traveling. On the left side of the model is the category of "sport tourism" where the primary reason to engage in travel is for sport purposes. Sport tourists may also engage in nonsporting activities, but this is a secondary intent or motivation for traveling. On the right side of the model is the category of "tourism sports" where the primary reason for travel is to engage in activities not related to sport. Nevertheless, these tourists also engage in sporting activities at some point during their trip. The two halves of the model are also delineated by hard and soft definitions. These hard and soft definitions further delineate tourists by the level of intensity and frequency with which they engage in the sport while traveling. Greater explanation of the model and various examples are offered below.

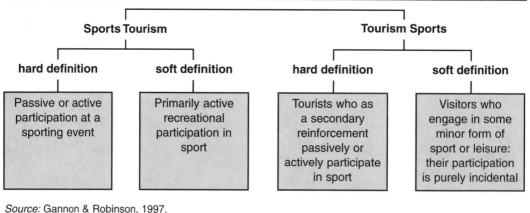

Source: Gannon & Robinson, 1997.

Figure 1.2. Sport and Tourism

Sport Tourism

Hard definition. These sports tourists travel outside their usual environment for the *primary purpose* of active (participant/organizer/official) or passive (supporter/spectator) engagement in a *competitive sport.* Examples of sports tourists who fit the hard definition would include a discus thrower traveling to the Olympics, an official traveling from England to Scotland to referee a soccer match, or the fan following the Australian cricket team to the West Indies.

Soft definition. These sport tourists travel outside their usual environment for the *primary purpose* of active (participant/spectators) engagement in a *recreational sport.* Examples of recreational sport tourists could include

- The enthusiast who takes a winter break in Florida to play golf;

- People who travel to the Columbia River Gorge to observe windsurfing at its best;

- A husband and wife who plan their summer vacation around rock climbing at Joshua Tree National Park, in California.

Tourism Sports

Hard definition. These tourists travel outside their usual environment for the *primary purpose* of engaging in *activities other than sports,* but they will actively or passively engage in sports as a secondary activity. Examples of people engaged in a hard definition of tourism sports could include

- People who travel to the Adirondack Mountains, New York, to see the natural beauty but who also try snow skiing

- Conventioneers who are in Miami for business but who also find time to watch a jai alai game at the local fronton.

Soft definition. These tourists travel outside their usual environment for the *primary purpose* of engaging in *activities other than sports,* but they may actively or passively engage in sports on an incidental basis. For example, when visiting Christchurch, New Zealand, to see its English-influenced architecture, a tourist decides to row a boat down the Avon River, or a sunseeker in Rio de Janeiro happens to play volleyball on the beaches after being invited by other people.

Sport-Event Tourism Model: Supply and Demand

Getz (1998) offers a third model of sport tourism that connects the supply side of the sports tourism industry with the demand side. In the middle of the model are tourism intermediaries who are the "connecting tissue" of the sport tourism industry. Intermediaries link the sport tourist with the event or destination in a variety of ways. Intermediaries are typically organizations that create sporting events to attract tourists, or they help organizations lure events to their destinations. In these roles, intermediaries are oftentimes convention and visitor bureaus or other types of organizations that contract out their services to help attract sporting events. In most cases, these organizations work with other intermediaries who supply travel and hospitality for the tourists. These organizations are tour operators, travel agents, tour wholesalers, and travel companies. Other types of intermediaries are the communications organizations that communicate the opportunities to the tourists by advertising or promoting events and activities.

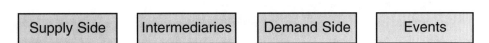

Figure 1.3. The Getz Model

On the demand side of the Getz (1998) model are the people who are likely to travel to the destination for sporting purposes. The governing bodies of sports, teams, individual participants, officials, spectators, and the media must all be "lured" to the event or activities. Given that each of these groups has different motivations and seeks different benefits through attendance, the suppliers and intermediaries must market and promote to the segments differently. On the supply side of the model are the event or activity organizers, hospitality services, and local media and participating sponsors. These entities are responsible for organizing a package of activities, attractions, and services that will be sufficiently enticing to cause people to travel.

Intensity of Involvement in Sport Tourism

Our model of sport tourism relates to the level of intensity with which people are involved in sport tourism. This model is purposely simplified to describe the hierarchy of intensity with which various groups use or serve the sport tourism industry. Although many factors play a part in ranking the intensity of involvement, the model serves to delineate between those people who are heavily involved in sport tourism and those who may have peripheral interest.

Demand Side: The Sport Tourist

The demand model is presented from the perspective of involvement of sport tourists in the event, contest, or competition, and possesses several dimensions. One is based on primary involvement (active participation); another, on secondary involvement; and a third, on spectator involvement (tertiary participation).

At the core of the concentric circles are those people who are most involved in the physical execution of the sporting activity and who are most needed for the activity to occur. This essential need also places these people in a category of the greatest intensity for demanding sport tourism services from suppliers. These people are the tourists who travel to the sporting activity as athletes, competitors, or participants depending on whether the event is competitive or recreational. These sport tourists are located at the inner core because they are most needed for the sport and for sport tourism to occur. Typically, they have the greatest intensity of involvement in the sport.

Some might argue that athletes cannot be considered sport tourists because for them the activity is not pure leisure behavior (freely chosen for intrinsic reasons and without obligation) and that pure leisure is at the heart of tourism. For the purpose of our discussion, individuals who travel for sport involvement, regardless of their motivations, are sport tourists.

In the next concentric circle are travelers who are actively involved in the sport but not playing the sport. These people are officials, organizers, statisticians, coaches, and trainers. The sport activity could take place without them although rarely does this happen. If it did occur, it would probably change the sporting activity from a competitive activity to a recreational activity. These individuals have the second greatest need for sport tourism suppliers because their involvement is usually necessary and the intensity with which they engage in sport tourism is strong. Usually, event organizers, officials, and coaches outnumber the participants so they have a wide circle to denote greater numbers. A caveat must be made with these types of sport tourists. It is debatable whether they are less intense about the sport they choose when compared to athletes, but it must be reiterated that the sport could continue without them, although at a less intense level.

Within the third ring of the demand side are spectators and supporters. Although their involvement and intensity can be very strong, these travelers are confined to an outer ring because they are not essential for the activity to occur. In many sporting events, the absence of spectators would cause financial ruin for the event. Spectators usually constitute greater numbers than do people in the inner circles because the former represent more of the general populace. These individuals demand the services of sport tourism suppliers but may also have alternative activities that draw their attention, interest, time and money. Because of their competing interests and needs, the third-ring travelers are harder to

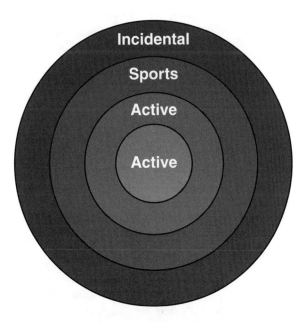

Figure 1.4. Demand Side Sports Behavior

attract to a sporting event than are those in the inner circles, but the spectators and supporters offer the greatest potential for profit.

There is a fourth ring of sport tourists. These people travel to the destination for other leisure-related purposes but attend a sporting event for a supplementary or incidental activity. Some of these people may visit the destination because the primary attraction is sport, but they are more involved with the pageantry and spectacle of the event than with the event itself. In this circle, the demand of sport tourism services is lowest because these travelers have many options from which to choose and their compulsion to attend is not as great. Although they may demand sport tourism services in advance, they are more likely to demand the services on the spur of the moment.

Supply Side: The Sport Tourism Supplier

In this part of the model, involvement in supplying sports tourism services is the key factor. As the concentric circles move outward, the suppliers of goods and service become less involved with sport tourism and more involved in meeting the demands of nontourists who need their services.

Participants in the sporting activity are both demanders of sport tourism services and suppliers of the same. Without their participation, other people would have no one to organize, officiate, support, or observe. Sport participants occupy the core, as they are an integral part of the supply side. There are other attractions that occupy the core beyond the athletes, and they may include sport museums, halls of fame, stadiums, sport speakers, instructors, natural sport challenges, and various human-made attractions.

In the next ring of the supply model are organizers, managers, promoters, and marketers of sport tourism opportunities. These people have direct involvement in the production of the sporting attraction and serve as the link between the sport and other tourists. At this level also are the sport organizations and associations, sport commissions, and local, regional, and national ministries of sport, which maintain the status of the activities on a year-round basis.

In the third concentric circle are the tourism suppliers, such as tour operators or travel agents, who get the tourists to their destinations. They also supply accommodations and culinary choices in packaged deals. These suppliers also offer the same services to other types of tourists. Given this dual focus, these suppliers occupy an outer ring because they do not focus entirely on either sport or sport tourism.

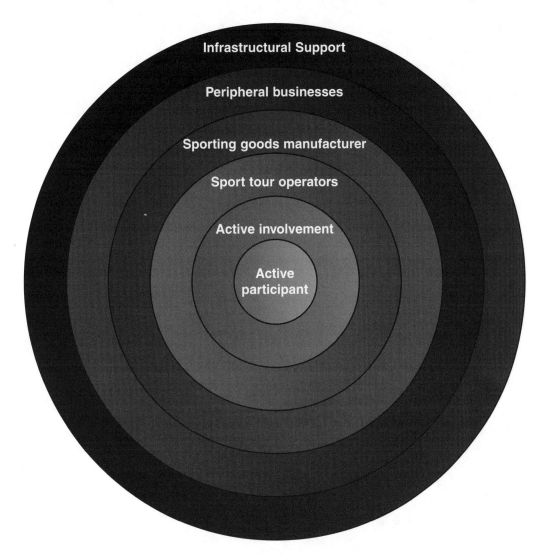

Figure 1.5. Supply Side Sports Behavior

At another level, but servicing everyone from the participants to the observers, are sporting goods manufacturers and retailers who make and sell equipment, apparel, and sports memorabilia. In some instances, these suppliers are also the primary or secondary attractions, especially if their factories or stores are set up as tourism attractions. Although these businesses are sport suppliers, they are less involved in the tourism business than are those individuals in the inner circles. Their aim is to sell goods rather than to promote travel opportunities.

At the next level of supply are the peripheral businesses that have a sport theme or a sport relationship. It is likely, however, that much of their revenue is generated by clientele who are not sport tourists. In this sense, the themed restaurant, hotels, eating and drinking establishments, concessionaires, vendors, and security all supply the industry but typically do not depend on its operation for the majority of their revenue.

At one of the outer circles is a very important supplier for sport tourism, but it is a small part of the many services they offer. It is here that local, state, regional, and national governments play a part. These entities provide infrastructure, such as roads, airports, utilities, and health and safety services. Governments provide policy and planning support as well as financial assistance to many events. Various levels of government may provide and maintain the natural resources where many sports are conducted. These natural resources can include rivers, seas, beaches, lakes, mountains, and forests, to name a few.

Now that the various models of sport tourism have been discussed, it is necessary to take a more comprehensive look at sport and tourism. To this end, the following discussion focuses on a definition and description of sport, whereas the next section describes the entire tourism system of services.

The Multiple Dimensions of Sport

Defining *sport tourism* is difficult because defining *sport* is equally difficult. Herein lies the problem. Is it considered sport when people load canoes onto their cars, drive to the local river, and take a Sunday afternoon float for five or six miles? Is it sport when the same people do the same thing, but they participate in an organized race with timing, prizes, and rules? Likewise, is it sport if people go to the local basketball courts for a pickup game, or is it sport when their team plays in a league every Thursday night. For that matter, are tractor pulls, darts, camel racing, or chess considered to be sports? When does sport become a sport, and when is it considered a recreational or leisure activity?

From a sociological viewpoint, Coakley (1998) states that "sports are institutionalized competitive activities that involve vigorous physical exertion or the use of relatively complex physical skills by individuals whose participation is motivated by a combination of personal enjoyment and external rewards." (p. 19). A competitive-oriented definition like this one eliminates the recreational canoers and the pickup basketball players. Therefore, it is important to examine the definition of sport and how this interfaces with sport tourism. The recent addition of competitive ballroom dancing as an Olympic sport fits nicely into Coakley's definition. It is institutionalized and competitive, and it involves very vigorous physical activity and complex physical skills. The dancers can also be motivated both extrinsically and intrinsically. If one observes ballroom dancing, one will see dancers who must be proficient in a variety of dance forms. These dancers are judged stringently by a group of officials and by comparison with their competitors. After ballroom dance competitions have been observed, it is apparent that dancing is physically demanding and that it requires strong motor skills, coordination, and endurance. Dancers can engage in dancing for pure enjoyment, but they can also be rewarded financially. Is ballroom dancing a sport?

The institutionalization of a sport refers to situations where the activity takes on widely recognized commonalties in terms of the way the activity is structured and understood by all those people who engage in it. For example, soccer is probably the most widely played sport in the world and is played the same way across borders and continents. Typically, the core of any sport is understood through the development of commonly used rules. Not only are rules commonly understood, they are also predetermined and codified into rulebooks of procedures, guidelines, and specifications. The governing organizations have developed these rules through a long process of regulatory evolution. Organizations are also the ones that control the contests, games, and competitions. Variations in the widely recognized rules do occur, usually to facilitate the sport for different age and ability groups. For example, beginning soccer has fewer rules than international soccer does so children can learn the general structure of the game. Commonly used methods of conducting the sporting episode also have variations depending on the situation. Basketball can be played indoors or out, and games can be played on large or small courts with high or low hoops. Although using the same methods as those of men's basketball, the women's collegiate and professional game in the United States has adopted a smaller ball to accommodate the smaller hand size of its competitors. Although basketball has a common core of understanding, the organizations that regulate, facilitate, and promote the sport also place their own variations on the game. To facilitate a better entertainment spectacle, the NBA professional game is longer, does not allow the use of zone defenses, and has smaller keyholes to allow post play closer to the hoop.

The second key word in Coakley's (1998) definition relates to the competitive nature of sport. Individuals, groups, or teams compete against other teams, groups, or individuals. They can also compete against standard measures such as time to completion, points awarded, particular accomplishments, or achievement of a goal that others cannot reach. The ultimate purpose in these competitions is to outdo the opponent in terms of points (lesser or greater) when the opposition is trying to stop or beat the individual, group, or team. In some situations, points are accumulated with no opposition. Contests always precipitate a hierarchy among the competitors, from more successful to less successful.

The third component of the definition is the phrase, *vigorous physical exertion* or *complex physical skills*. These terms are incomplete, leaving undetermined how vigorous *vigorous* is or how complex *complex* is. Could the sport of fly-fishing be considered vigorous? It is certainly not as vigorous as ballroom dancing. Nevertheless, many people call fly-fishing a sport. Many people also call chess a sport, but the vigorous nature is more intellectual than physical. It may well be that vigorous involvement is a better term than vigorous activity, but certainly for most sports, physical activity is a necessary entity to its engagement.

The final part of the definition encompasses the rewards, benefits, and motivations for engaging in sport. Sports can be done for intrinsic satisfaction. That is, the sport is enjoyed for its own sake or for the inherent pleasure that is derived from engagement. On the other hand, sports can be extrinsically satisfying, too. Sport might be engaged in to receive recognition from other people, to interact with friends, or to receive payment for the activity being undertaken. Inevitably, the rewards or benefits are a combination of both although one might wane in favor of the other. The professional softball player may have started the sport as a child for the pleasure of playing, but later in a professional career, he or she may play more for the financial reward than for the inherent pleasure the game brings. Part of the complication of defining sport motivation is the professional element. When does the professional sporting activity cease to become a sport and begin to be more of an entertainment extravaganza? Is professional wrestling a sport, or is it entertainment?

Coakley's (1998) definition of sport seems far too limiting for the purpose of defining sports tourism. To include recreational sports such as hunting, chess, or canoeing, the definition offered by Coakley must be altered. In the altered definition, the sport person engages in an activity that has been formally recognized as a sport, but he or she may have little need for the formal rules, regulations, and boundaries that come with institutionalization. In our definition of sport as it relates to sport tourism, the activity must be formally recognized as a sport, but it need not have the accou-

---

What is your definition of sport?

Is it related to the more traditional definition that encompasses rules, competition, and physical activity, or does it extend to recreational activities undertaken by people during their leisure that are not controlled by these factors but can be controlled by these factors under the right circumstances?

Which of these activities would you consider to be sport?

Professional Wrestling	Hunting	Chess
Jet Skiing	Fishing	Frisbee
Bungee Jumping	Competitive Ballroom Dancing	Skydiving

trements of playing within the rules and regulations. Furthermore, competition is not necessary, and outward physical exertion need not be observed even though many sport tourism events have this component. For our definition of sport, the activity need only be regarded as a sport. The way it is conducted need not be physical or competitive.

What Is Tourism?

After defining sport, it is also necessary to define *tourism* and *tourists*. Although a sociological definition of tourism producers could be provided, an economic definition suits sport tourism more readily because most tourism services involve a purchase-for-service exchange. From a supply-side orientation, tourism is better defined from a business perspective.

A tour is a trip that returns to its place of origin and is derived from the Latin *tonare* and the Greek *tornos,* which signifies a lathe or a circle, the movement around a central location. The "ism" is defined as an action or a process and, in this case, the process of leaving and returning to the same point. With "ist," as in tourist, the suffix refers to a person who undertakes a particular action or function. Thereby, the tourist is a person who engages in the process of leaving and later returning to the same point.

Until a few years ago, a singular definition of tourism did not exist. Many businesses, governmental units, and organizations defined tourism in different ways for their own purposes. In 1991, the World Tourism Organization (WTO) organized the International Conference on Travel and Tourism Statistics to address the problem of common definitions. They had the intent of creating one set of definitions that could be used worldwide. By creating common definitions, used all over the world, the number of tourists, the dollars spent on tourism, the lengths of stay, and the jobs generated could be measured in a standard manner. Only when this standardization was complete could the magnitude of tourism be fully described. Although far from complete, the first stage of defining tourism and tourist is now in place.

With over 90 countries represented, the conference decided on a common set of definitions for both domestic and international travel, and on a system that categorized tourists into commonly recognized economic classification units. When tourism activity was organized into accounting systems used by countries, the economic activity and impact could be measured. The tourism definitions listed below are the results of the 1991 conference held in Ottawa, Canada.

Tourism: "activities of a person traveling to a place outside his or her usual environment for less than a specified period of time with a main

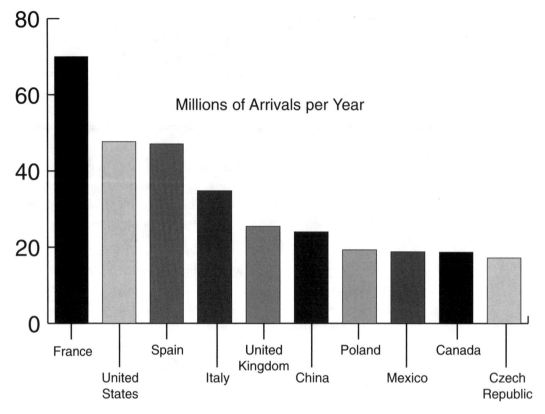

Millions of Arrivals per Year

Figure 1.6. Top 10 World Destinations

purpose other than the exercise of activity remunerated from within the place visited (World Tourism Organization, 1991, p. 3)." To further understand this definition, its key terms are discussed below:

- the "usual environment" was meant to exclude trips within the place of residence and routine trips such as traveling a long way to and from work on a daily basis;

- the "less than specified period of time" was meant to exclude long-term migration such people who travel to another country to live; and,

- the "exercise of an activity remunerated from within the place visited" was meant to exclude migration for temporary work.

This broad definition was preferred by the conference so that it would identify the activities of tourism within a country and between countries. Until recently, domestic tourism has been regarded as being less important although statistics typically show that domestic tourism is much larger than international tourism in most countries of the world. The encompassing definition of tourism was further broken into three subcategories: domestic, national, and international. In the discussion that follows, maps indicate the different subcategories:

Domestic tourism. This comprises "internal tourism and inbound tourism, where internal tourism refers to residents of a country visiting their own country, and inbound tourism refers to visits to a country by non-residents" (WTO, 1991, p. 4). Domestic tourism, in the diagram below refers to tourist activity within the United States, whether the tourists are U.S. citizens traveling within the United States or foreigners coming to and traveling within the United States.

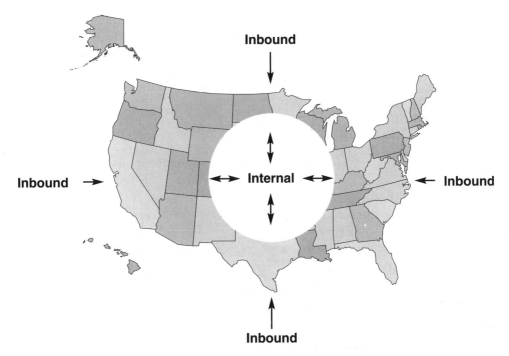

Figure 1.7. U.S. Domestic Tourism

National tourism. This comprises "internal tourism and outbound tourism, where outbound tourism refers to residents of a country visiting other countries" (WTO, 1991, p. 4). National tourism, in the diagram below would refer to tourist activity within the United States by U.S. citizens or United States citizens who travel outside the United States to visit other countries.

International tourism. This subcategory "consists of inbound tourism or outbound tourism" (WTO, 1991, p. 4). International tourism, in the diagram below, would refer to all tourist activity that crosses the borders of the United States. See figure 1.8.

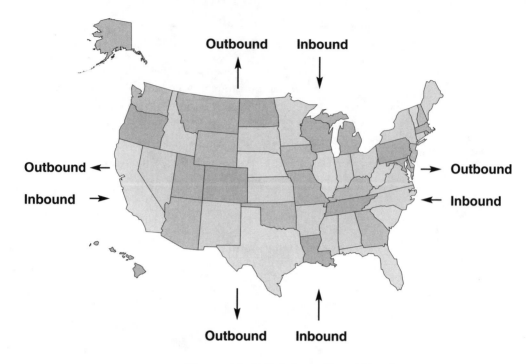

Figure 1.8. U.S. International Tourism

After defining tourism, the World Tourism Organization (1991) conference went on to categorize the people who engaged in the tourism. When making these categorizations, the WTO needed to delineate between the place of residence and the type of traveler based on length of time away from home and length of stay in the destination the traveler visited. Listed below are the descriptions of a resident, visitor, tourist, and same-day visitor. The conference also saw the need to separate these travelers by the type of tourism they were undertaking, international tourism or internal tourism. Therefore, there are two descriptions for each of the four categories:

1a. Resident (International): "A person is considered to be a resident in a country if the person has lived in that country for at least a year or twelve consecutive months prior to the person's arrival in another country for a period not exceeding one year."

1b. Resident (Internal): "A person is considered to be a resident in a place if the person has lived in that place at least six consecutive months prior to the person's arrival in another place for a period not exceeding six months."

Interpretation. It was necessary for the WTO to define where people traveled before they determined if they were a traveler. The key differences be-

tween the two descriptions included traveling to another country (International) and traveling to another destination in the same country (Internal). In these cases, residency requirements and the time away from home were shortened by half for the internal travelers. The thought behind the shortened residency requirements and shortened stays was related to the ease with which one can change residences within one's own country. If it is easier to move residences, then stays away should also be shorter before the traveler becomes a resident of another place within that country.

2a. Visitor (International): "a person who travels to another country other than that in which he has his usual residence for a period not exceeding one year and whose main purpose of visit is other than the exercise of an activity remunerated from within the country visited."

2b. Visitor (Internal): "a person residing in a country, who travels to a place within the country, outside of his usual environment for a period not exceeding six months and whose main purpose of visit is other than the exercise of an activity remunerated from within the place visited."

Interpretation: *The difference between the two descriptions is related to the visiting of another country and the visiting of another place within the same country—the times have been adjusted accordingly. In addition, the visitor's main purpose cannot be to earn money in the place visited.*

3a. Tourist (International): "a visitor for at least one night but not more than one year and whose main purpose of visit is other than the exercise of an activity remunerated from within the country visited."

3b. Tourist (Internal): "a visitor for at least one night but not more than six months and whose main purpose of visit is other than the exercise of an activity remunerated from within the place visited."

Interpretation: *Although the differences of within and outside the country still exist, to be classified as a tourist, the person must stay overnight in the place visited, whether it is internal travel or international travel.*

4a. Same-day visitor (International): "a visitor for less than 24 hours and not involving an overnight stay in the country visited and whose main purpose of visit is other than the exercise of an activity remunerated from within the country visited."

4b. Same-day visitor (Internal): "a visitor for less than 24 hours and not involving an overnight stay in the place visited and whose main purpose of visit is other than the exercise of an activity remunerated from within the place visited."

Interpretation: *As a same-day visitor, the person stays in the destination for a very short time. The international same-day visitor may be a cruise* *passenger where the boat only stays during the daytime. This kind of traveler may also be a person who has crossed international borders to witness, officiate at, or engage in a sport but who returns home after the contest is over on that particular day. Internal same-day visitors may have traveled to a sporting event, within their own country, for the day, but they return home after the event is over. (WTO, 1991, p. 5–6, Sect. 3). In both cases, receiving money from the place that is visited cannot be the primary reason for traveling to the destination.*

Overall, all the people in the definitions are travelers; however, many people who are travelers may not be included in tourism statistics. When traveling internally and internationally, there are several travelers who are not considered tourists. Internal travelers who are not tourists can be

- People temporarily or permanently moving their residence

- People admitted to institutions for long-term stays but with no intention of residing there

- Military people on maneuvers

- Nomads

- Commuters who travel outside their place of residence

- People who engage in travel within the bounds of their residential area.

International travelers who are not tourists include

- People who cross an international border every day to work

- People who are temporarily or permanently moving their place of residence

- Nomads

- People in transit lounges awaiting their travel connection

- Refugees

- Armed forces members

- People who work in foreign offices abroad and diplomats.

Chapter 2

The Sport Tourism Industry

Questions

1. What are the components of the sport tourism system?
2. What are the problems in providing sport tourism services and how may they be overcome?
3. What are the consumer motivations for sport tourism?

Introduction

Now that we have defined sport and tourism, it is time to explore the workings of the sport and tourism industries. The sport tourism system will then be considered with regard to the broader tourism industry. In addition, the reader will be introduced to some basic motivations of sport tourists and the benefits of sport tourism in general.

The Sport Industry

The sport industry is defined as the market in which the sport products and services are offered to buyers. Pitts, Fielding, and Miller (1994) identified three segments in the sport industry, labeled (a) sport performance segment, (b) sport production segment, and (c) sport promotion segment. In their model, the aforementioned segments were further delineated by product and buyer segmentation variables. As a product, sport performance is offered to buyers who are participants or spectators. As a participation product, sport performance is offered to the buyer in various forms and means. Consumers may select any number of sports, settings, skill levels, and market segmentation offerings (e.g., gender, age divisions). As a product for spectators, sport is offered through personal attendance at an event or via the popular media. Although experiencing sport through the popular media can stimulate subsequent travel, experiencing the sport as a nonresident is the purest form of sport tourism; the tourist as participant or as spectator.

Within the sport production segments are products and services necessary or desired to produce sport or to influence the level of sport performance (Pitts et al., 1994). To be performed, many sports require certain products. For example, in the production of a hockey game, a participant needs skates, a stick, goal, and puck. In an officially organized competition, one would also need a hockey rink and referees.

The sport promotion segment comprises those goods and services used in the promotion of the sport to its interested publics. Some of the contributing components to the sport promotion segment are enterprises involved in television production and broadcasting, Internet information, magazines, newspapers, and countless advertising and public relations outlets.

Other peripheral services for sport tourists include lodging accommodations, travel agents, eating and drinking places, and transportation providers. Support businesses for sport tourism include concessionaires, vendors, security, telecommunications, and logisticians. Direct infrastructural support includes that provided by local, provincial, state, national governments, transportation, utilities, and health and safety services. Government[s] may also provide financial resources, planning, and policy assistance to the sport tourism industry. For many sports, natural resources serve as the foundation upon which the sport tourism industry is based. Natural resources also serve as an attraction for the mountain climber in Nepal; the mountain biker in Moab, Utah; and the downhill skier in Thredbo, Australia.

The Sport Tourism System

The sport tourism system differs little from regular travel and tourism systems except that its destination attractions are focused on sport activities. This system, depicted in Figure 2.1, is very similar to tourism systems previously advanced by Gunn (1988) and Mill and Morrison (1992) although it recognizes politics to be at the center of the system.

The tourism system is a delicate system. It is highly dependent on the economic health of sport tourists to provide revenue and of the national currencies they use. Sport tourism is also a volatile business environment because many companies form alliances to gain market advantages and many other companies go in and out of business.

Governmental politics can change the nature of the tourism system with a policy change as can fare wars, different promotional campaigns, new and competitive technologies, and new attractions. In addition, the tourism system is delicate because many components of the system are designed to serve residents and tourists alike. They do not exclusively serve one or the other. With competing demands, suppliers may not serve either as well as they could if they were exclusive. With competing demands, moreover, suppliers may choose to concentrate on one particular client group while ignoring the other (Gunn, 1988).

The sport tourism system is divided into six components, with a seventh being added for differentiating between primary and secondary attractions. Between most of the main components are links that assist with the function of the main component. Only one component fits on the demand side of the sport tourism system, which is composed of the potential sport tourists or the consumers. These are the individuals who want to travel for the primary purpose of sport: participants, officials, organizers, and spectators. The following section will describe each component of the sport tourism system.

CONSUMERS—The process of buying a sport tourism experience is a complex one. It is affected by countless variables that individuals never consciously consider but that affect their decisions. Much of the buying decision is shaped by motivations, attitudes and constraints on travel. The sport tourism consumer process is important, and these factors are listed and discussed below.

Consumer Process When Purchasing Sport Tourism

1. The consumer's *attention* is directed to sport tourism attractions.

2. The consumer gathers *knowledge* about various options.

3. *Personal attitudes/interests* as well as skill level mediate the intensity with which each option is considered.

4. *Evaluations/Preferences* by the consumer serve to eliminate or rank available options.

5. Even though the consumer *intends to buy* the sport tourism preference, it may not happen.

6. The sport tourism option is *purchased.*

In the realm of sport tourism, much of what sells relates to consumers' interests and motivation, but it also relates to the amount of information they have about their options. It is here that information supply,

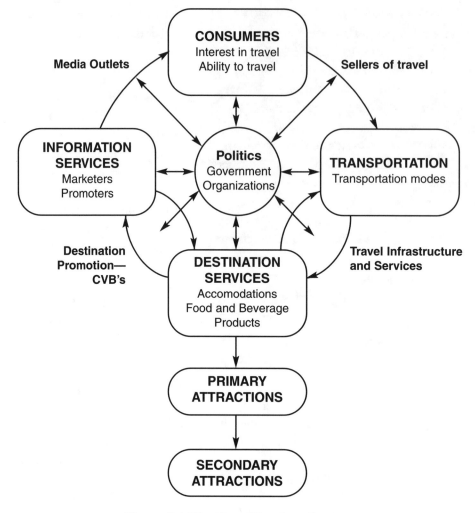

Figure 2.1. The Sport Tourism System

promotions, and the media are very important. If the potential sport tourist is unaware of opportunities, he or she will never choose to visit a destination or a sporting event. Getting the *attention* of the potential sport tourist is a major step. Consider that consumers, on average, are bombarded by over 2,500 advertisements per day in various forms (Assael, 1987). If the promotional efforts are successful when catching the attention of individuals, potential sport tourists usually need more *knowledge* about the destination and the sport tourism opportunities. Because travel is personally risky due to its large costs, a great deal of knowledge needs to be accumulated. Potential sport tourists will also want to know time frames for traveling, costs, accommodations, experiences to be gained, and many other details regarding the trip. This knowledge must appeal to the sport tourists' needs and wants so they feel that they will be receiving the benefits they desire. Potential sport tourists will also want to know about other options so they can choose the best option. After the knowledge has been gained, the next step depends on how potential sport tourists feel about the sport tourism options. In this sense their *attitude and interest in* the opportunity will help predict their propensity for traveling. For example, a person may be attracted by the media attention given to the ESPN Extreme Games. However, after finding out where the Games will be located and gathering information about the various events, costs, and destination, that individual does not explore the opportunity further because his attitude toward the Extreme Games and interest in the Games is not strong enough to continue. If the attitudes and interests are positive, then an *evaluation* of the sport tourism opportunity must be conducted among many competing opportunities. The option that is evaluated most positively will determine the sport tourism choice.

With the destination and sporting attraction decided, the sport tourist has the *intention* of traveling to the destination. This intention may be counteracted my many competing factors, such as lack of time, money, or sport tourism opportunities that come along later. If these factors are surmounted, then the tourist may *purchase* their trip (Assael, 1993; Mill & Morrison, 1992).

Although the sport tourist's decision-making process may seem simple, it is complicated by many steps before the actual travel episode takes place. How many times have people expressed an interest in traveling to a particular place only to recant their positive expression at a later date? Sport tourists must have not only a willingness to travel but also the ability to travel after they consider the opportunities and constraints they face.

On the supply side of the tourism system are the other components. Essentially the supply components are all those below the consumer component on the diagram. Each of these will be discussed in a clockwise rotation around the system.

Travel intermediaries are the organizations that bridge the gap between the consumer and organizations that supply the transportation, hospitality, and attractions services. The travel intermediaries' role is to develop, advise, and book travel services for travelers. They are called intermediaries because they do not provide the service, but they assist people in accessing services from suppliers of air travel, accommodations, and attractions. Because these linking or intermediary agencies do not produce the services such as accommodations, travel, or attractions, there is less incentive for them to promote particular places. They are more likely to sell what they think consumers will buy and what the consumers request from them. Discussed below are some of the main types of travel intermediaries, such as tour wholesalers, tour operators, retail travel agents, and electronic intermediaries.

Tour wholesalers package transportation, hospitality services, and attractions into one saleable item that is made available to the public. Typically, the wholesalers do not deal directly with the public, but they make their packages available through retail travel agents and other intermediaries. These wholesalers buy transportation services, hotel rooms, food and beverage services, and attractions in bulk from suppliers. In return, they receive a bulk discount, some of which is passed on in savings to the consumer. That is why purchasing packaged travel is typically cheaper than buying the components of travel separately. The "waters are muddied" in the tourism wholesaling business because retail travel agents, tour operators, and travel companies are now compiling their own packages and selling them directly to consumers. Many of these wholesale packages are targeted to specific types of consumers, such as sport tourists, but they may also feature particular destinations (Indianapolis Speedway), types of transportation (train rides), types of activities (outdoor pursuits), and special interests (sports card collecting).

Wholesalers put together three main types of travel packages, depending on the needs of targeted clients and the types of activities to be undertaken. *Escorted travel packages* use professional tour guides who travel with the group through the entire tour and who organize the details of the tour en route. Sometimes these guides offer instructions and commentary about the activities and destinations encountered, and other times they handle logistics only. *Hosted travel packages* are group tours that are greeted and accompanied by hosts in each destination, but the hosts do not make the entire tour with the group. The last type of tour is a *package tour*, which is a collection of transportation, accommodation, and attractions without escorts or hosts. Packaged tours are structured to allow travelers more freedom to do what they wish in particular destinations.

The next type of intermediaries is the *tour operator*, who strictly handles the logistics and operations of the tour. Once tour operators have organized the travel, they let other organizations market and sell the package before providing the service. Tour operators may be an airline or a bus company.

Retail travel agents are the most visible travel intermediary for the buying public because they have stores located near travelers' residential areas. They advertise, sell, and reserve tours, vacation packages, airline tickets, hotel rooms, car rentals, cruises, and other services needed by the traveler.

For the reservation and sale of services, retail travel agents receive a commission that is a percentage of the cost. In most cases, retail travel agents are travel counselors trying to fit the best travel plans to the traveler's needs. In the past, consumers did not pay extra for the counseling services as the agents received their money from the travel suppliers. More recently, commissions from suppliers have been reduced, and many travel agents have started to charge additional fees for their services. With commissions being cut, travel suppliers selling directly to the public, the growth of Internet travel booking, and the consolidation of travel agencies into national corporate conglomerates, the number of retail agents is falling. Clearly suppliers of travel services would rather not pay retail agents, so suppliers are findings ways to cut agents' commissions.

Although there are many other types of intermediaries for the sport tourist, the newest type is predicted to grow dramatically. *Internet travel services* are becoming more popular because travel consumers can book their own transportation, accommodations, and attractions by searching on the Internet. Web sites such as Travelocity, ITN, and Expedia are becoming more popular as people familiarize themselves with computer technology and Web site offerings. These sites usually link with the computers of travel suppliers and list their offerings and prices for consumers. The key benefit for the consumers is that they can develop their own itinerary and services at the prices they choose. The benefit for Web site providers is that they do not have to pay commissions to travel agents because each reservation comes directly from the consumer. Even more recent than the aforementioned Web sites are other sites where consumers can suggest a price they would like to pay for a hotel or airfare. Travel suppliers can then choose to accept the offer or not. The

- Two-thirds of the 90,000,000 U.S. travelers were on-line
- 59,000,000 used the Internet to plan for travel
- Sixty-nine percent of frequent travelers use the Internet to plan for travel
- Twenty-seven percent (27%) of travelers on-line used the Internet to make travel reservations—an increase of nearly 60% since 1999.
- Thirty-seven percent (37%) of Internet users planned vacations on-line
- Forty-six percent (46%) of Internet users planned automobile vacations on-line
- Forty-one (41%) of Internet users planned air travel trips on-line
- Sixty-percent (60%) of Internet users searched for maps and directions on-line
- Fifty-three percent (53%) of Internet users searched for lodging on-line
- Forty-one percent (41%) of Internet users searched for airfares/schedules on-line

"Searching" on-line does not necessarily mean purchasing on-line

Figure 2.2. Internet Usage by American Travelers—2000

benefit of these sites is that consumers can suggest what they are pre-pared to pay whereas travel suppliers can accept the offer if they have an empty airline seat or hotel room. www.Priceline.com is an example of one such travel service provider. If suppliers have strong demand for their services, they can ignore the offer, but if demand is low, they can accept the offer and fill their vacant slots.

The *transportation* sector of the tourism system is devoted to organiza-tions involved in moving people for travel and tourism purposes. Air-lines, cruise ships, bus companies, trains, and rental car companies provide the majority of these services although most tourism is still un-dertaken in private motor vehicles. The mass transportation methods listed above are called *common carriers*.

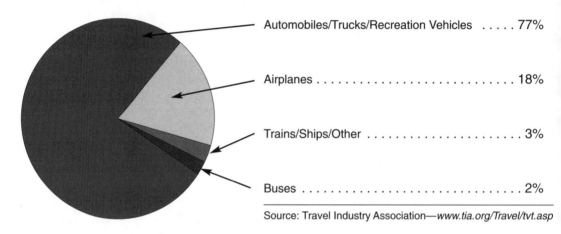

Source: Travel Industry Association—*www.tia.org/Travel/tvt.asp*

Figure 2.3. Transportation Methods of U.S. Travelers—2000

There are several factors related to how people choose a mode of trans-portation, but the most prevalent factors are convenience and cost. The following sorts of concerns determine whether a person will choose her own motor vehicle or a common carrier.

- Does the carrier leave from and arrive at convenient locations when compared to the traveler's needs?

- Does the common carrier leave and arrive at convenient times?

- Is the common carrier physically convenient to use?

- Is the distance traveled more convenient for motor vehicle use or a common carrier?

- Is the cost of a common carrier congruent with what the traveler is prepared to pay?

When based on the grounds of convenience, it is not surprising that the large majority of sport tourism is undertaken in private motor vehicles although this decreases as distance traveled increases. Other factors may also enter into transportation choices. For cruises, part of the attraction relates to the services received onboard and the relaxed nature of the travel. For exotic transportation modes, such as sailboats or supersonic aircraft, a novelty and prestige factor is included. The most prominent types of common carriers are airlines.

Airlines. Airline travel has changed significantly since the Wright Brothers' first flight over 100 years ago. Much of the airline travel today is due to technological advances that have made airline travel cheaper, airplanes larger, and reservations easier. It is also due to the 1978 deregulation of the airline industry in the United States. Prior to deregulation, particular airlines were authorized to fly particular routes under a governmentally controlled pricing system. With deregulation, many airlines were permitted to offer flights on a free-market basis and charge

Table 2.1. The Largest U.S. and International Common Carrier Airlines—2000

Rank	Carrier Name	Country	Traffic (Billions of RPKs*)
1.	United Airlines	US	201.9
2.	American Airlines	US	180.1
3.	Delta Airlines	US	168.6
4.	Northwest Airlines	US	119.3
5.	British Airways	UK	117.4
6.	Continental Airlines	US	96.6
7.	Air France	FR	85.5
8.	Japan Airlines	JP	84.3
9.	Deutsche Lufthansa	DE	81.4
10.	US Airways	US	66.9
11.	Singapore Airlines	SG	65.7
12.	Qantas Airways	AU	59.9
13.	KLM Royal Dutch	NL	58.9
14.	Southwest Airlines	US	58.7
15.	All Nippon Airways	JP	56.7
16.	Trans World Airlines	US	41.9
17.	Cathay Pacific	HK	41.5
18.	Air Canada	CA	39.0
19.	Thai International	TH	37.6
20.	Alitalia	IT	36.8

*Revenue Passenger Kilometers = paying passengers multiplied by distance traveled
Source: http..../prome/8-INTERNATIONAL-AIRLINE-UPDATE—The-World—140-s-air-carriers.htm.

prices based on market strategies. Many new airlines entered the business, but most experienced financial demise. Today, apart from low-cost carriers such as Southwest Airlines, the major carriers use a hub-and-spoke system of smaller planes bringing passengers from regional airports (the spokes) to major airports (the hub) where travelers transfer to larger planes for longer flights.

Although the hub-and-spoke system has proven more efficient than previous methods, some low-cost carriers have forced the major carriers to fly direct commuter flights to serve business travelers. The major airlines also fly internationally. It is here that they face more competition because some foreign airlines are subsidized by their governments, whereas American airline companies are not. In many other countries of the world, regulations do not permit competitive practices, and the costs for passengers are high.

For sport tourists, airlines offer the advantages of quick long-distance travel at reasonable rates to almost anywhere in the world. Added to these national and international common carriers are charter airlines that schedule flights on request, when passenger loads are sufficient to make it profitable. Also added into the mix of airline companies are regional carriers. It is typical for these regional carriers to have agreements with large airline companies. They carry passengers on the spoke flights feeding the large carriers for the long flights.

Cruise lines. Cruise ships and cruise lines have enjoyed a renaissance from the days when the primary role of an ocean liner was to transport people between continents. The primary routes of cruise lines today include the east and west coasts of the United States, the Caribbean islands, around the European subcontinent, including the popular Mediterranean cruise routes, and Southeast Asia. Nowadays, cruise ships do not stop at several ports to pick up their passengers. They most frequently depart and return to the same port with passengers being flown into that port as a part of a packaged airfare. In the future, we may see marketers using the term *voyage* rather than *cruise* to describe this tourism experience.

Sport-related cruises are primarily themed events where enthusiasts travel on particular ships that have contracted with sports stars to lecture and mingle with the passengers. Niche markets are also being formed in various sports although cruise lines are increasingly stocking their cruises with sporting equipment and with sports-related excursions in each port of call. The Norwegian Cruise Lines, for example, recently advertised a variety of sport cruises where the attractions are not ports but the sports themes onboard. These themed cruises were pro basketball,

Cuervo Gold Untamed Volleyball, Diet Coke Champions of Fitness, pro baseball, *Sports Illustrated* Afloat, and Motorsports Cruise Rally ("Advertisement," 1998).

Coach transportation. Bus companies in the sport tourism business are typically chartered for specialty trips or group tours. Many of the bus companies have entered the tour operations business for themselves, creating sport package tours so they can fill their buses. The decline in the number of regular bus passengers made this change of strategy necessary. The number of regular bus passengers diminished when private motor vehicles became ubiquitous. Sport tourists who use bus tours are those in large groups with relatively short distances to travel. Bus travel then becomes more affordable and convenient when compared to individual cars or airlines. Bus travel is also a preference for people who like to have all their arrangements taken care or for those who fear flying.

Rental cars. The majority of car rentals occur after tourists reach their destination. After disembarking from an airplane, they use rental cars to move around the destination. Although business travelers dominate the weekday market, leisure travelers dominate the weekends. Given this orientation to rental car use, it is not surprising that much of the rental car travel market emanates from airports.

Rail transportation. Train travel has faded in the face of competition from private motor vehicles and airplanes. Trains have very little flexibility to move where the demand is greatest, so rail passengers are faced with slow, long-distance travel to predetermined locations around the country. When competing against other long-haul transportation such as airlines, trains are too slow and have little variety in terms of destination choice. When operating against shorter distance transportation options, trains cannot compete with the door-to-door convenience of private cars. Although train travel has declined in the United States, it is very popular in countries where people own fewer private vehicles and automobile ownership is expensive. In these countries, trains run their routes more frequently and to many destinations, which makes them more convenient to use. The train trip is an important part of the full leisure experience, providing opportunity for spirited anticipation and socialization, as evidenced by train travelers to football matches in the United Kingdom.

Infrastructural travel support consists of organizations and agencies involved in the supply of infrastructure for moving people around. Many times this infrastructural support is governmentally supplied and funded by taxpayer money. It is here that airports, docks, roadways, utilities, safety services, and transition points fit into the sport tourism system. If

Table 2.2. Twenty Busiest Airports in the World 2000

Rank	Airport	Country	Total Passengers
1.	Atlanta, Hartsfield	USA	80,171,036
2.	Chicago, O'Hare	USA	72,135,887
3.	Los Angeles Int'l	USA	68,477,689
4.	London, Heathrow	U.K.	64,607,185
5.	Dallas/Ft. Worth	USA	60,687,122
6.	Tokyo, Haneda	Japan	56,402,206
7.	Frankfurt	Germany	49,360,620
8.	Paris, Charles de Gaulle	France	48,240,137
9.	San Francisco	USA	41,173,983
10.	Amsterdam, Schiphol	Netherlands	39,604,589
11.	Denver	USA	38,748,781
12.	Las Vegas, McCarran	USA	36,856,186
13.	Seoul	Korea	36,727,124
14.	Minneapolis/St.Paul	USA	36,688,159
15.	Phoenix, Sky Harbor	USA	35,889,933
16.	Detroit Metro	USA	35,535,080
17.	Houston, Intercontinental	USA	35,246,176
18.	Newark	USA	34,194,788
19.	Miami	USA	33,569,625
20.	New York, J.F.K.	USA	32,779,428

Source: http.//news@airwise.com/airports/frame/2000top50.htm.

the infrastructure is complete and developed, travelers do not notice it. However when roads are bad or waiting lines at borders and airports are long, frustrated tourists experience considerable vexation. The development of proper infrastructural services not only benefits the sport tourist, but it also benefits everyday citizens who reside in the travel destination. The most obvious types of infrastructural development are airports.

Destination services comprise suppliers who offer accommodations, food, beverages, entertainment, and products. When one considers accommodations, one typically thinks about hotels. However, accommodations can also include resorts, campgrounds, motels, bed-and-breakfast units, and a variety of dormitory arrangements. Sport tourists most often use hotels because they are the most prevalent forms of accommodation. A hotel was once defined as an establishment that offers rooms only, with the possibility of restaurant services included. Today, hotels also offer many other services, including pools, fitness areas, and shops. Hotels are most often located in areas where a lot of business is conducted or at transition points in travel (e.g., near airports). They are located in these places to take advantage of people staying away from their usual place of residence. Hotels can also be found in places where there are continuous attractions, such as those linked to convention centers or stadiums. Resorts differ from hotels because they are usually designed with more leisure in mind and for longer-stay patrons. The prime differences between resorts and hotels include locations in scenically attractive places and the variety of recreational activities they provide. Resorts may also be located close to natural resources where people like to engage in outdoor sports or leisure. Participatory sport tourism is linked to resorts with sport facilities serving as the primary attraction (e.g. golf, tennis, swimming). Motels are the other common variety of accommodations. They are typically located by infrastructural routes such as highways to house travelers on-the-move. Motels tend to be cheaper and tend not to provide services found in hotels or resorts. Similar to hotels, motels are transitioning into a variety of services. Varieties in pricing can be found within all of these accommodation choices.

- Budget accommodations offer basic rooms and relatively inexpensive food.

- Midrange accommodations offer more in-room luxuries and a variety of eating choices at more expensive prices.

- Luxury accommodations have many room and service luxuries with fine dining available. The variety of food and beverage establishments is endless, but it is worth knowing the variety of meal plans that may be included in accommodation prices:

- European plan—no meals included in accommodation prices.

- American plan—three meals per day included in the accommodation price.

- Continental plan—continental breakfast included in the accommodation price.

- Modified American plan—two meals per day (usually breakfast and dinner).

While discussing food and beverage services, it is important to note the availability of sports bars and restaurants. Each sports bar or restaurant may be related to a particular sport or sports figure, or may cover all major sports. Examples include Shoeless Joe's in Chicago (named for the infamous Chicago White Sox player), the Toronto's SkyDome restaurant, and the old Ponsonby "Pot," a pub in Auckland, New Zealand, that serves as a haven for rugby players and fans. More recent themes are being established in bars and restaurants, including the ESPN Zone, that use electronic media to relay a variety of sports. The patron may be seated in front of the screens that broadcast their sport.

The *primary attractions* of sport tourism are the activities that lure tourists into participation, organization, or spectatorship. If the attractions meet tourists' expectations, they also provide the primary source of satisfaction. These sport attractions may have continuing activities, or they may be intermittent. In the sense of being continuous, the sporting attraction may be activities that can be engaged in year round. Such would be the case for windsurfing in the Caribbean or competing in 10-pin bowling. Other types of year-round sporting attractions are the places where the sport is celebrated but not played. Sport bars, restaurants, halls of fame, and museums are those attractions that most easily come to mind. Many sporting events are limited by season or by athletes' need for "down time." These attractions will be seasonal or intermittent. Other sporting attractions could be termed periodic rather than regular. Mega-events usually fit this category and would be characterized by the NBA Finals, the World Cup of Rugby and Soccer, the America's Cup, and the Olympics.

Besides considering the regularity of the sporting attractions, consideration must also be given to the setting in which the attraction is conducted. Attractions in natural settings rely upon the elements of the environment to play an integral part in the sporting activities. The activity relies on the natural environment to provide much of the challenge. Activities that characterize this type of attraction may be hang gliding, surfing, or rock climbing. These types of sporting attractions must be contrasted with events, such as soccer, that are played outdoors but on surfaces prepared by humans to enhance the game. Sporting attractions where the natural environment is not integral to the activity can be labeled *human contrived*. Human-contrived attractions can be broken into two subcategories. The first are the settings such as fields and stadiums designed specifically for sport and spectatorship. The second are those settings designed to "reproduce" sport. The sporting activity is not conducted at the location but is reproduced through pictures, televisions, and memorabilia. In all of these environments, a participant may compete against a standard, against external forces, or against other people.

Natural Resource-Based Sporting Attractions
Against nature and external standards—canoeing, rock climbing, windsurfing
Against nature, standards and competitors—triathlons, windsurfing races, orienteering

Table 2.3. Secondary Tourist Attractions

Natural or Scenic	Human Contrived	Historic	Cultural/Ethnic
Beaches	Airports	Battlefields	Antiquities
Canyons/gorges	Amusement/theme parks	Birthplaces/famous people	Archeological sites
Caves	Antique shops	Burial grounds	Art galleries
Cliffs	Arenas/stadiums	Historic buildings	Ceremonial displays
Climate	Art galleries	Ghost towns	Costumed events
Desert	Beauty spas	Historic tours	Early settlements
Fall foliage	Botanical gardens	Landmarks	Ethnic celebrations
Fishing streams/lakes	Bridges	Memorials	Exhibits
Forests	Campgrounds	Missions	Mansions
Geysers	Churches	Monuments	Museums
Islands	Crafts shops	Museums	Native crafts/culture
Lakes	Dams	Old forts	Prehistoric items
Mountains	Dude ranches	Pioneer places	Re-creations/restorations
Nature trails	Entertainers	Reconstructed historic places	Special events
Ocean	Farms, ranches	Reenactments	Trading centers
Picturesque views	Ferryboats	Ruins	Unique lifestyles
Rivers	Gambling		
Sand dunes	Harbors		
Swamps	Health resorts		
Unique geologic sites	Night clubs		
Valleys	Orchards/vineyards		
Volcanoes	Parks		
Waterfalls	Planetariums	**Other Recreation Activities**	
Wildlife	Playgrounds	**Special Events**	
	Ships		
	Shopping		
	Shows		
	Ski slopes		
	Swimming pools		
	Theaters		
	Wharves		
	Zoos		

Source: Adapted from Mill, R.C. (1990*). Tourism: The international business.* Englewood Cliffs, NJ: Prentice Hall.

Human-Contrived Attractions

Against contrivance—indoor rock climbing, recreational golf
Against others in contrivance—Lacrosse, soccer, rowing, luge

Human-Reproduced Attractions

Education and Entertainment—sport museums, bars and restaurants, sport card shows, stadium tours

Secondary attractions are usually tourist attractions that have little to do with sports. They provide alternatives for the individual interests and fill in time between sporting activities. With several types of attractions (including sport) in one area, the tourist destination has a much better chance of succeeding. A variety of attractions will lure a variety of people, and they will be attracted over a greater number of months. Variety will also help to lure tourists back for things not done on previous visits. The types of secondary attractions are voluminous, but presented below is an incomplete list.

Destination promotions encompass the variety of information suppliers located in the tourist destinations. They spread the word about their attractions with the goal of bringing in visitors. These promotional suppliers can include convention and visitor bureaus, sport associations, regional and national tourism promotion boards, sport leagues, and individual sport teams. The intent of these information suppliers is to provide information that will catch the attention of sport tourists. They provide further information so those potential visitors can build their knowledge base about the destination. In some cases, these suppliers will help with packaging trips to their location. All the aforementioned entities use similar methods to attract tourists:

- Advertising—paying to distribute information and catch awareness through television, magazines, brochures, newspapers, the Internet.

- Publicity—using newsworthy events to catch distribute information and catch awareness through their coverage by various media entities.

- Public relations—promoting a good public image for the sport tourism destination.

- Incentives—enticing tourists with competitions, awards, deals, and packages.

- Convention and visitor bureaus (CVBs) work on behalf of citizens and businesses to attract visitors. Through the efforts of CVBs, money is infused into the community through tourist spending. As stated by Newman, "a bureau brings hotels, restaurants, shops, attractions and a host of other businesses together into a single enterprise dedicated to sustaining and improving the travel and tourism in its community" (1993, p. 3). When visitors are enticed to a destination, the CVB should provide contacts and reservation assistance for accommodations, transportation and attractions. Many CVBs work in conjunction with local sport commissions to attract, bid to host, and retain sporting events.

Information services are suppliers who spread the knowledge of sport tourism opportunities to all potential consumers. The usual media are television, the Internet, radio, newspapers, and magazines. This information may be developed by travel writers, tourism promotion boards, trade magazines, newspapers, brochures, and sport or travel trade shows.

Politics are in the middle of the tourism system because they affect all aspects of sport tourism. In sport tourism, the political players can include many organizations, but they also include interpersonal and interoffice politics. The following entities are involved in the political dimensions of sports tourism:

• Sport organizations and associations establish the rules of engagement and conduct for participants and fans alike. They determine who can participate and where the participation will occur. For example, the International Olympic Committee is very politically involved when establishing who can be involved in the Olympics and where they will be held. Each time an individual or country is banned, there is a political outcry, and each time they choose the next Olympic venue, politics are involved. Consider the scandal surrounding the Salt Lake City, Utah, bid to host the 2000 Winter Olympic Games and the subsequent policy changes and restructuring of the IOC in response to the political outcry.

• Local, regional, and state governments regulate travel and tourism because they control and fund infrastructural necessities. Without the support of the state, Utah's roads, airports and accommodations could not have been expanded for the Winter Olympics and funding would have been impossible.

• National and international regulatory organizations develop rules to govern travel. Thousands of international rules govern travel, and among them are determinations on where planes can fly, who can get visas, how money is exchanged, and how payments are made for travel.

• Countries will often govern where and when their people can travel, and sometimes, how much they can spend while outside the country. The country may also discourage its citizens from visiting particular places.

Sport tourism is also governed by political ideologies. The United States and several other governments withdrew from the Moscow Olympics in 1984 to protest the invasion of Afghanistan. Although terrorists have attacked two Olympic Games to dramatize their political causes, sport has also been used to heal political wounds and promote ideologies. For instance, the United States and China used Ping-Pong diplomacy to thaw the Cold War between them, and wrestling was used to promote dialog between the United States and Iraq. The "sport machines" that produced athletes in East Germany, U.S.S.R., Cuba, and China in the 1960s and 1970s were used to showcase the achievements and superiority of Communism.

Furthermore, boxing matches in the 1970s such as the "Rumble in the Jungle" and the "Thrilla in Manila" were used to enhance the international profile of Uganda and the Philippines respectively.

The four areas in which governmental control is most evident are promotion and subsidization, legal controls, regulation, and safety. Included here are some instances where this happens to airlines and airline operations. In subsidization, most governments subsidize their airlines because they are too expensive to run privately. Through tax breaks, cheap loans, and cash payments, governments support their airlines. With regard to promotion, almost every country has a national tourism promotion board that bespeaks the benefits and attractions of their country. These boards are funded by monies provided by their governments. The legal controls are developed so that tourism organizations will operate as legal and ethical businesses. In the case of airlines, each airline must abide by its obligation to carry passengers at the times advertised and to offer reparations when they fail, as dictated by market forces. Finally, there are the rules of safety, which in the United States are controlled by Federal Aviation Administration. This agency regulates airspace, issues licenses to pilots, and judges the structural integrity of airplanes. In air travel, many trade associations also oversee their members to make sure that rules and regulations are followed.

Perhaps the largest impact of politics is applied through the granting of passports, visas, and other controls of movement between countries. In the United States alone, seven governmental departments control travel in and out of the country. Passports are granted to establish identities and places

Political Turmoil in New Zealand Sport Tourism

As with other segments of the tourism industry, sport tourism has its political influences. In New Zealand in the 1980s, the country was torn asunder by the imminent arrival of the South African national rugby team. The team had been denied travel by other countries because of the apartheid policy of its government. (Apartheid was a policy of separate development between the numerically dominant black population and the politically dominant but much smaller white population.) As controversial as this policy was, the New Zealand government, on the basis of hints of change in South Africa, decided not to put politics in the way of sport. It decided not to deny the South African team entrance visas, thereby allowing them to play rugby in the country. While the decision maintained the ruling party's political standing amongst its members, the country was torn apart by those who did not want politics in sport and those who thought that allowing the South African rugby team into New Zealand was a tacit approval of their apartheid and racist political agenda. In great secrecy and under heavy security, the South African team arrived. New Zealand protesters of the tour physically fought with New Zealand supporters of tour, sometimes dividing friends and families. In one of the early games in the province of Waikato and after several clashes outside the rugby stadium, protesters stormed through the fences and onto the field. After arriving on the field, the protesters distributed broken glass and nails on the field in hopes of canceling the game. With the field later cleared, the game could have taken place except for a lone individual who had stolen a light airplane and threatened to fly it into the main grandstand. The game was called off. Protesters fled, with several being severely beaten by rugby supporters. Into the night, vigilante squads of rugby supporters scoured the city in search of protesters and beat those they came across. It was just a game that ignited and inspired a quiet country to explode.

of residence. Visas are issued to establish the lengths of stay and the type of activities that can be conducted when visiting. In addition, travelers may need to provide information about their health and to pay taxes on goods brought with them.

Prior to democratization, the former Soviet Union restricted some of its athletes from participation in foreign contests for fear that, seeking political asylum, the athletes might defect to the host country. Similarly, Cuba, protective of its national baseball team, has determined the international contests the team may play according to the government's relations with the host country and the perceived threat of player defection.

It is now time to turn our attention to the difficulties with which the sport tourism system operates. Quite apart from the political machinations and the coordination of several industries into one, the nature of providing tourism services is very difficult on four counts. The following discussion examines those four counts.

Problems of Providing Sport Tourism Services

This system differs from other business systems that one might encounter. For example, if the system were designed to supply home computers, the goods would be manufactured and sent as close to the consumer as possible for ease of purchasing. In any tourism system, the attractions and many of the services are immovable and so the tourist must travel to the destination in order to consume them—the lived experience cannot be shipped to the consumer's home. This is a specific problem with all service-dominated industries, and it is not the only problem. Information widely available in services marketing publications indicates that service-dominated industries must deal with four main problems. However, the information in this study is largely based on the work of Lovelock (1984), Zeithaml, Parasuraman, and Berry (1990) and Berry and Parasuraman (1991).

Intangibility of Services

In a service-dominated industry such as sport tourism there are few products to be sold. One may argue that sporting goods are a part of the sport tourism industry, but when compared to the dollars generated in other sectors, the total amount is relatively small. What is being sold to the sport tourist, as in all tourism encounters, is an experience, something that is intangible. This intangible service may be providing the experience of observing a professional baseball game or the experience of playing in a chess tournament, but the sport tourist comes home with only memories. Even the hotel rooms and airline flights are mere memories after the event is over. Apart from photos, videos, and some memorabilia, little that is tangible carries over after the sport tourism service has been consumed. When experiences are being sold, it is hard for potential sport tourists to compare between offerings because they cannot try the experiences out first. In order to have the sport tourism experience, one must pay for it first and experience it later. When one buys a car, one can take many models for a test drive to determine the best one before purchasing it. After the purchase, the car remains as tangible evidence of the money expended. This places potential sport tourists at a great deal of personal and financial risk because they cannot be sure of the sport tourism service they are buying. They cannot be guaranteed that the experience will be worth the money they will spend.

There are several ways to make intangible services more tangible:

1. Make sure all the sport tourism providers are qualified with credentials that indicate a high standard of professionalism

2. Advertise the credentials and special skills of sport tourism service providers

3. Use celebrities to serve as spokespeople for the sport tourism service. If the service is good enough for them to endorse it may be good enough for sport tourists to purchase

4. Provide testimonials from sport tourists who have used the service previously

5. Provide a credible brand image that is recognizable to sport tourists. Consumers tend not to trust generic brands compared to recognizable brands

6. Make sure that all visual impressions of the sport tourism service provider are professional, including the ambiance of offices and the dress of workers.

7. Allow "test drives" if possible and if not, at least allow trials for intermediaries such as travel agents who can pass information by word-of-mouth

8. Conduct followup surveys of and phone calls to sport tourists so to reassure them that they are still valued customers and to find situations where they were dissatisfied with the service.

Inseparability of Production and Consumption

As stated before, to produce a sport tourism experience, the sport tourist must be present to consume it. The sport tourism experience is very difficult to manufacture in Sydney and send to the consumer in Rome. Because sport tourists must be present to produce and consume the experience (inseparability), they must always be brought to the site of the sporting activity. This creates an access problem for many tourists because travel and stays away from home are expensive. Television and the Internet have lessened this problem as sporting events can be broadcast to consumers. However, these consumers are not tourists and do not leave the financial benefits in the sporting destination.

There are several ways sport tourism marketers can reduce inseparability. Listed below are several marketing strategies:

1. Provide packages with many services for one price.

2. Attempt to develop sport tourism opportunities in geographically dispersed places such as may be found with high-adventure sport tourism companies that operate in the outdoors. REI offers outdoor sport tours through its many different and widely dispersed store locations in the western region of the U.S. For REI, there is a greater chance that one store location will be closer to the consumer.

3. Provide sport tourism opportunities in places where there are a variety of other attractions so that the site will attract many people in a group or family, not just sport tourists.

Perishability of Services

The third problem of the sports tourism service industry is that the sport tourism events (attractions) must go on as scheduled whether or not sport tourists arrive. There is a large loss of money to be dealt with if there are few spectators or few competitors or if airlines and hotels are empty. The event seats cannot be saved for another time and neither can the hotel beds—they will perish if not used when offered. When revenue is lost because of empty seats or beds, it is lost forever because the stadium seat that was unfilled yesterday cannot be saved and filled today. In addition, the sport tourism industry is often capacity constrained. If too many tourists arrive, it is very difficult to add seats to an airplane, rooms to a hotel, or seats in a stadium to serve them. Again, money is lost, and sport tourists may be dissatisfied.

Several ways exist to reduce perishability:

1. Offer differential pricing between peak seasons and off-peak seasons to disperse the bulk of sport tourists.

2. Provide reservations systems to guarantee availability of the services.

3. Educate sport tourists about off-peak times.

4. Provide plenty of peripheral services to engage sport tourists if the main attraction is busy or delayed.

5. Contract to other service providers when you cannot deal with the capacity.

6. Market to different segments in off-peak times with different sporting activities. For example, downhill skiing communities have marketed their areas to mountain bikers and extreme sport enthusiasts during late spring, summer, and early fall months in attempt to increase tourism volume.

Heterogeneity of Service Offerings

The final problem that sport tourism encounters is the heterogeneity or inherent changeability of service quality. If a manufacturer sells a product, the company can test it before they sell it. They can ensure its quality before it leaves their factory. When providing sport tourism services/experiences, the weather may be bad, the game may be boring, the hotel service may be inadequate, or the directions to the venue may be poor. In a service industry such as sport tourism, it is extremely difficult to guarantee a quality experience that meets and exceeds the needs of all consumers all the time. There are too many variables to control to make the experience perfect in all situations, and one small misadventure may diminish the total package.

Several actions may be taken to reduce heterogeneity:

1. Standardize as many of the components of the sport tourism experience as possible, especially if they are provided for mass consumption. Standardization will help guarantee better overall quality.

2. Customize sport tourism services when people want special attention, services, or experiences. For example, during the Indianapolis 500 some tourists require tickets to the race, while others demand access to time trials, museum tours, and pre and post race parties.

3. Concentrate on internal marketing so those employees providing the services do so at their peak ability and capacity.

4. Provide necessary training and repeat the training periodically so that employees continue to provide quality services.

According to Kurtzman (1997), the impetus for engaging in sport tourism can be divided into two sets of choices. In the first instance, sport tourists are not fully aware of the influence upon them when they

The Sport Tourist–Behavior and Motivations

decide to travel for the sake of sport. This *pseudo-choice* is the result of compounding forces, such as family, friends, peer groups, and media messages. The second type of choice is *intentional choice*, which occurs when the sport tourist has an internal affinity for sport and is moved to travel because of a liking for sport. These descriptions are somewhat limited, and so it is necessary to review other motivations.

The internal motivations of the three main types of sport tourists (spectators, organizers, and participants) are somewhat different. For the sport spectator, motivation may lie in the observation of sport as a way to express desires and interests. Spectators may also be motivated by being with others who enjoy the same sport or through a deep sense of commitment (fan) to the sport (Sutton, McDonald, & Milne, 1997). People who are working at a sporting event may have several different motivations. These people may reap monetary benefits from working a sporting event, such as being paid referees or officials. They may also be compelled to travel because of their official status or because they are officials with a competing team. For these people, their commitment is to the sport rather than themselves (Skirstad, 1996). Sport participants are motivated to travel for several reasons. They may be motivated to compete as a test of their preparation or to compete against others. At a less serious level, they may want to remain involved in sport because they enjoy the activity and socializing that accompanies it. Finally, one must not forget the motivation of money that is an inherent part of professional sports.

After viewing the motivations of people engaged in sport, it is also necessary to review the motivations of tourists. Crompton (1979) put forth a set of social psychological motivations for pleasure travel that have remained solid and accepted over time. *Social motives* relate to interactions with others whereas *psychological motivations* relate to individually held reasons. Crompton acknowledged that attractions are important motivations, but he also found that many motivations for travel do not relate to destination attributes. Crompton found 10 motivations that will be discussed in the context of sport tourism. Some of these motivations are *push factors* whereas others are *pull factors*. Push factors are reasons why people want to *get away* from their regular place of residence, and pull factors are reasons for *going to* particular destinations.

Push and Pull Factors

Escape from a perceived mundane environment. For many people escape from the constancy of everyday life is important. People are trying to escape not only their physical environments but also the obligations of jobs, home, and society. The old adage that "a change is as good as a rest" applies in this situation. According to Crompton (1979), escapism begins before the act of travel. The psychological anticipation of a trip is inherently releasing. Additional evidence suggests that people escape from both mundane environments and overstimulating environments (Iso Ahola, 1984). For example, a production line worker may use sports tourism to get away from the drudgery of work, whereas the commodity trader may use it as release from the stress of creating multiple deals.

Exploration and evaluations of self. People need to leave their regular environments to test themselves in different situations. Through sport tourism, this exploration and evaluation may be undertaken by competing against others or by competing against oneself. Other times they learn a lot about themselves and how they cope in unfamiliar settings. When traveling to a foreign country, sport tourists are compelled to negotiate languages, cultures, monetary exchanges, and social mores.

Relaxation. In Crompton's (1979) study, respondents talked about feeling physically exhausted after coming home, but also feeling relaxed. Even though they are physically exhausted, people can refresh themselves emotionally and psychologically by concentrating on activities that are different from those at home.

Prestige. Some people are motivated by the potential for enhancing their status. The prestige of a destination may be attributed to tourists in terms of increasing their status among peers. In part, prestige is a factor of exclusivity because few people have the opportunity to travel whereas the majority of people stay at home. Following this notion of exclusivity, Pearce (1988) suggested that greater distances provide greater exclusivity and higher prestige. Exclusivity may also be provided through sporting events that are difficult to attend. Attending the Super Bowl, mountain biking in Moab, Utah, or skiing in Aspen would fit this description admirably. Social desirability is the other important factor of prestige (Riley, 1995). A softball tournament in Antarctica may be exclusive, but it may not be socially desirable for other people. If there is no element of desirability, the travel will not be prestigious.

Regression. During episodes of tourism, people get to do things that are different from their usual routine. In the case of regression, they relive past behaviors and activities. "Dream" baseball camps where adults can participate in spring training workouts with former athletes is one example of a sport tourism experience targeting those who long for the days not only when they played the sport but also when their favorite players were on their favorite team. Reliving old behaviors is easier when traveling because the attitudes and norms of one's home environment are not constraints.

Enhancement of kinship relationships. Tourism can be a way of bonding with one's family. At home, family members have their own agenda, but during tourism, people are linked by a single theme. This theme may be a father and son viewing a soccer game or a mother and daughter playing in a fast-pitch softball tournament.

Facilitation of social interaction. Meeting other people was found to be a tourist motivation. Sometimes the contacts are fleeting, but at other

Table 2.4. Personality Types and Travel Propensities

Allocentrics	*Psychocentrics*
Lifestyle/Personality	**Lifestyle/Personality**
Nonrestricted lifestyles	Restricted lifestyles
Outgoing	Inhibited
Confident	Lacking confidence
Feel in control	Sense of powerlessness
Adventurous	Unadventurous
Travels for business	Works close to home
Travels for pleasure when able and can afford	Travels when necessary or obliged
Inquisitive	Not inquisitive
Try new products and services	Does not try new products or services
Moderate to high risk-takers	Low risk takers
Media Consumption	**Media Consumption**
Light television watcher	Heavy television watcher—comedies
Prefers newspapers and magazines	Reads few magazines
Tends to watch pro football	Tends to watch baseball
Likes television documentaries	
Resources	**Resources**
Upper income levels (top 5%)	Lower income levels
Use disposable income	Withhold income(saver)
Travel Preferences	**Travel Preferences**
Travel to areas not frequented by tourists	Travel to familiar places
Like to see and do new things	Like to see and do familiar things
Destinations that are different	Sun & fun destinations, relaxing
High activity	Low activity
Like to fly to destinations	Like to drive to destinations
Less developed hotels, services, attractions	Developed hotels, services, attractions
Foreign people and cultures	Familiar people and cultures
Little organization, maximum flexibility	Complete tour packaging

times, travelers are looking for more permanent relationships. According to Crompton (1979), the best way to fulfill this motivation is through living in accommodations that are close and attending events where there is a common denominator. Sport is a common interest for many, and the subject of conversation between tourists and residents of the host community. It would also seem that people traveling alone are more likely to interact with others than are people who travel in groups. Solo travelers look outward whereas groups spend their time maintaining solidarity.

Novelty. The novelty motivation refers to people who travel for new and exciting experiences. Some travelers will always seek these experiences whereas others are inclined to return to the same destination every year.

Education. Some travelers perceived the education motive as a moral imperative. To visit a destination without learning something was viewed as wasteful.

Beyond travel motivations are personality types that mediate the propensity to travel. It is here that Plog's (1972) research shed some light on why particular individuals are more adventuresome than others. When researching nonfliers, Plog found different types of travel personalities. The three main types were *Allocentrics*, who were very adventurous; *Midcentrics*, who held a middle ground; and *Psychocentrics*, who were very inhibited in their travel. Although Midcentrics constitute the majority, we can more easily understand the propensity if we consider the two extremes. In general, it was found that people with more resources, education, and confidence were also the more adventurous tourists. People with lower resources, education, and confidence tended to stay much closer to home. Allocentrics were more likely to travel to exotic places whereas Psychocentrics were more likely to follow their local sport team. Table 2.4 shows the characteristics of the two groups.

Sport Tourism as a Distinct Market Niche

Why should sport tourism be the focus of further study and the subject of this book? The reasons are several, but one of the undeniable reasons is that sport is pervasive in society.

- First, there is increased access to sport via increased supply from sport providers and the awareness generated by popular media sources.

- Second, there is increased access to sport for segments of the population who were underserved, including women and girls, minorities, and individuals with disabilities.

- Third, substantial gains in per capita discretionary income have increased access to sport for most segments of the population. Finally, sport has been elevated to a level of social and cultural prominence in society.

Increased Sport Access to Society

Sport has increased access to consumer markets because of increased coverage from popular media. We have also become more aware of numerous sport destinations and attractions via mass information systems. Today, it is difficult to avoid the variety of television programs, newspaper articles, specialty magazines, and radio shows that send a sport-based message. There are also more financial benefits and opportunities for sport participants and entrepreneurs than there once were. Increasingly, sports are becoming more accessible through greater organization at the amateur level and greater variety at the professional level. Furthermore, sport is more open and inclusive to segments of the population previously excluded from participation. In the United States, the effects of Title IX for women, the Americans with Disabilities Act, and the Paralympic Games are some of the examples of greater inclusion when compared to historical examples. Enacted in 1972, Title IX of the Civil Rights Act requires educational institutions to provide equal sport and recreation opportunities for women and girls. Better physical health of older adults has allowed for their sport participation later in the human life cycle. It is not uncommon to see retirees who follow a trail of golf courses or older adults who participate in cross-country skiing at various sites. We are a more mobile society. People now have greater access to mass transportation than ever before. The notion of geographic distance has been diminished by modern transportation systems. Increased discretionary income has allowed many people to negotiate the financial constraints associated with sport tourism.

Sport Prominence in Society

Sport has been elevated to a level of prominence within and beyond cultural contexts. To our society, sport is becoming equal to or more central than other established institutions, such as religion, family, government, and education. Turco and Eisenhart (1998) described the growth in sport as a focal attraction:

Sport participation and attendance have become a global phenomenon and international sports competitions have fueled an ever-increasing world tourism market. International competition in soccer, track and field, tennis, yachting, golf, and the Olympic Games have vastly increased spectator interest, stimulated nationalism, and to some degree broadened intercultural perspectives that all benefit the tourism industry.

Sport is a contemporary way of anchoring oneself within a culture when many traditional anchors have disappeared. It is also a way of identifying with other people across cultures. It has become easier for one to say, "I am a Green Bay Packer fan" than "I am a Lutheran." It may also be easier to start international diplomacy with Ping-Pong or wrestling than it is to argue the issues of difference. It is in sports where nations that are apparent enemies might find common ground.

Sport tourists tend to be more involved in their chosen attraction than do sightseers of the traditional visual attractions. This heightened involvement may be due to the significance of the sport or contest beyond alternative cultural, social, and economic opportunities. The sport, the team, the sports star, or the sporting culture the sport tourists follow may be more important than their job, their community, their school, or their religion. These institutions provide an external structure by which they must abide, but sport provides an activity in which they may or may not participate.

Sport also provides opportunities for involvement where the consequences of involvement are less severe. It is here that the sport fan can enjoy themselves for their own sake rather than for the sake of long-held tradition and law. For example, the Field of Dreams in Dyersville, Iowa, has a meaning to tourists

Sport Tour: Cape Town, South Africa

The tourism and sport industries in South Africa have not reached their full potential in terms of economic development, largely due to the apartheid policy of the former political regime. The 1970s witnessed the onset of serious political and social instability as a result of apartheid. The end to apartheid and the country's first democratic elections in 1994 had a dramatic effect on overseas tourism. The World Tourism Organization (WTO) now considers South Africa one of the most promising tourism destinations on the African continent. Sport tourism has a strategic role in achieving the aims of the Reconstruction and Development program that aims to uplift South African society economically. Capetonians and South Africans generally are passionate about sport. For several years, two events unique to Cape Town, the Two Oceans Marathon and the Argus Cycle Tour, have attracted thousands of visitors to Cape Town annually.

The Castle Lite Two Oceans Marathon is a spectacular 56-km road race along the scenic Cape Peninsula, which attracts about 10,000 competitors from all over South Africa. International interest has been growing since 1992. The Argus/Pick 'n Pay Cycle Tour draws 28,000 entrants to Cape Town who participate in a grueling 105-km race around the Peninsula.

However, only recently has Cape Town begun to realize the contribution that sport tourism can make toward a sustainable tourism industry. Cape Town hosted the opening ceremony of the 1995 Rugby World Cup. This event marked the return of South Africa to hosting major sport events. Furthermore, the Rugby World Cup and the 1996 African Nations Cup of Soccer demonstrated the capacity of major sport events to be significant nation builders in creating, peace, goodwill, and understanding in South Africa.

The bid for the 2004 Olympic Summer Games presented Cape Town with an opportunity to market itself as a world-class city. Although Cape Town did not win the right to host the Games, benefits gained during the bidding phase included the roofing of the Belleville Velodrome, which provided the venue for the 1997 World Junior Cycling Championships. The bidding further catalyzed the construction of an international-standard softball stadium as well of three multipurpose indoor halls in previously disadvantaged areas. As a result of this process, Cape Town and South Africa are seeking ways to further develop the tourism product of South Africa through the sport tourism segment of the industry (Government of South Africa Tourism White Paper, 1996).

beyond the sport of baseball. It enjoys a cult-like following due in part to the movie's popularity and the nostalgia associated with the period depicted in the movie. It conjures up a feeling of a simpler, purer time in America for visitors to the site. The Major League Baseball Hall of Fame in Cooperstown, New York, is a historical sport attraction that represents the collective meaning of baseball history and culture. Similar to the Field of Dreams, the Baseball Hall of Fame is visited by African-Americans to understand the history of the Negro League as representation of their struggle for acceptance and eventual inclusion in U.S. society. The Baseball Hall of Fame's exhibit honoring the Ladies Professional Baseball Association, popularized by the movie *A League of Their Own*, has a similar effect on female visitors. In South Africa, a national sports museum has recently been established with the aim of teaching South Africans about their sporting past and providing inspiration for the future.

There are other location icons associated with sport that attract tourists even when the sport is not taking place. Visits to attractions, either primary or secondary in motive, are made by sport fans to the All-England Tennis Club in London, which hosts the Wimbledon Tennis Championships; the Indianapolis 500 Motor Speedway; and Lambeau Field, home of the Green Bay Packers of the National Football League. For the sports fan, such sites serve as tangible, enduring symbols of their sport, team, or star when other tangible anchors have diminished.

Unique Characteristics of the Sport Tourism Markets

The study of sport tourism is important for several reasons. One can be a sport tourist for most periods of the life cycle. A sport tourist can be a 5-year-old participating in a regional youth gymnastics meet or a 95-year-old competing in the Senior Olympic Summer Games. The individual or group nature of sport tourism also warrants investigation. One can be a sport tourist as an Australian surfer along the coast of Thailand or as a member of the New Zealand "All Blacks" rugby team on a tour of South Africa.

There are many ways in which one can be involved in the sport tourism industry. A sport tourist can be either actively or passively engaged through sport participation or spectatorship. One can be a sport tourist as a cricketer in Pakistan or a cricket match spectator at the Melbourne Cricket Ground in Australia.

Sport Tour: Green Bay, Wisconsin

The Green Bay Packers of the National Football League (NFL) provide a unique case example of the influence sport can have on a host community. The Packers have played before 185 consecutive sellout crowds at Lambeau Field, dating back to 1960. The capacity of Lambeau Field is 60,790, including 2,702 private box and 1,920 club seats. Local businesses have benefited by the Packers' recent success on the playing field. In 1997, the Green Bay area's 3,065 rooms were sold out the weekend of Super Bowl XXI, even though the game was played in New Orleans! Mike Kanz, director of the Green Bay Convention and Visitors Bureau, estimated the impact of the preseason training camp on the host economy to be $4 million, double the revenues of the previous summer.

The tourism influence of the Green Bay Packers is felt in community 30–40 miles away. During a regular season weekend, a Green Bay home game fills over 75% of the 2,331 hotel and motel rooms in the Appleton area, 30 miles southwest of Green Bay. In 1997, 39 lodging establishments totaling 3,338 rooms were sited in Brown County, 198% over the 1980 room totals. Local lodging accommodations were booked full during home game weekends, with most hotels/motels requiring a 2-night minimum stay. Lodging sales tax revenues for Brown County in 1996 totaled $37,879,703, up 5% from 1995 ($36,195,606). For 2 weeks following the Super Bowl XXI victory, telephone inquiries to the Green Bay Area Convention and Visitors Bureau increased 500%, with two thirds from out of state. Located next to the team's training facility and the Green Bay Packers Hall of Fame, the Packers Experience is an interactive event that challenges participants to pack, kick, run, block, and do the Lambeau Leap.

The stadium is also tourist attraction when it is empty. More than 29,000 visitors toured Lambeau Field in 1996. The status of the event and the novelty/appeal of the sport attraction and host community may influence upwards the spending behaviors of sport tourists. It had been 30 years since the Green Bay Packers of the National Football League (NFL) had participated in the Super Bowl before their appearance in 1997. The novelty of their appearance in the title game, coupled with the abundant hospitality and entertainment options available in New Orleans, triggered an unparalleled level of spending among Packer fans worldwide. Sales of Super Bowl XXXI merchandise, most of it featuring the Green Bay Packers, hit a record-setting $130 million. In 1996, sale of licensed Packers merchandise was 5.6% of the total among the 30 NFL teams. In 1997, it was 14%. In January 1997 alone, Packers merchandise sales totaled $70 million. Attendance at the Green Bay Packers Hall of Fame in 1996 totaled 160,607, up 65% from 1995. A $1,040,000 expansion of the Packer Hall of Fame was completed in 1997 in response to increased visitor volume. The image of the city is intertwined with the team. Packerland Drive, Lombardi Avenue, and Holmgren Way are examples of transportation arteries in Green Bay named after the team and its Super Bowl-winning coaches. Similarly, the names, promotional messages, and decor of numerous local businesses reflect strong identification with the team.

Chapter 3

Making Dollars and Sense: Economic Impacts of Sport Tourism

Questions

1. How is the economic impact of sport tourism defined?
2. What are the economic costs and benefits of sport tourism?
3. What are the various methods to estimate sport tourism economic impacts?
4. What is the multiplier effect and its relationship to sport tourism economic impacts?

Introduction

Economic impact is defined as the net change in a host economy directly attributed to a sporting event or operation. There are four primary considerations when assessing the economic impacts of sport:

1. The extent to which the sport stimulates new spending within the economy,

2. The extent to which the sport retains local income,

3. The costs to produce the sport, and

4. The extent to which the economy internalizes spending attributed to the sport.

This chapter describes the economic costs and benefits of sport tourism and methods to assess sport tourism economic impacts.

Economic Impact　Economic research has been previously conducted on such diverse sport tourism events as auto racing (Burns & Mules, 1989); professional football (Regan, 1991); hot air balloon championships (Turco, 1995); and the Olympic Winter Games (Ritchie & Aitken, 1984). The economic impacts of conducting a sporting event and investing in sport facility development projects, and of tourists' expenditures on sport participation and spectating may be categorized as primary or direct impacts. *Direct impacts* arise from transactions closely related to the event, such as material and labor purchases made when expanding recreation facilities or the expenditures for various supplies and services for event participants and spectators. *Indirect or secondary impacts* include the chain of events that result from the direct effects, including changes in employment levels, gross regional product, factor earnings, and institutional incomes like personal income or government revenues. Nonmonetary benefits such as increased awareness and enhanced image of the host community are also considered secondary impacts of a sporting event. The geographic origin and ultimate destination of spending attributed to sport tourism operations have significant influence on its economic impact.

Spatial Distribution of Sport Tourism Spending

The spatial nature of sport tourists attraction spending can be best understood by dividing it into impact regions. Direct economic effects are geographically distributed throughout an economy because sport tourists often make purchases during various phases of their trip. Purchases are made at home in advance of the trip, en route, at or near the sport site, on the return trip, and at home upon return. Indirect effects are likely to take place far from the location of direct effects due to the interregional industry linkages. An economy may import goods and services from many areas, thereby scattering portions of the direct sport tourist transaction across the globe.

To illustrate the spatial nature of sport tourist attraction spending, a conceptual model of impact regions is featured in Figure 3.1. The smallest spatial unit is the sport attraction site, the physical location of the attraction. This may include the sport stadium, arena, natatorium, or other sport venues. Expenditures occurring within this region are typically made for purchases of food, beverages, entertainment, and gifts/souvenirs. Although total on-site expenditures may be considerable for large-scale attractions, they are often less significant than the economic activities occurring in other regions.

Many of the direct economic impacts of sport attractions occur in the second region, "support area." The primary objective for defining the support area is to identify the sectors of the economy most affected by tourism expenditures. Businesses typically affected by tourism include those that provide lodging, eating and drinking, and transportation.

Data required to accurately measure sport effects within and outside a designated economy must clearly distinguish income retained (and continuing to circulate with an economy) and income "exported" by identi-

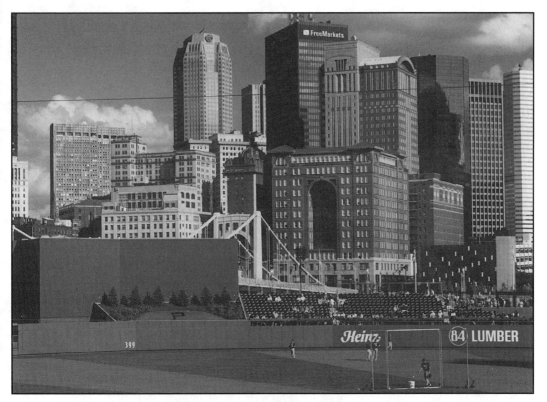

While sport tourists may come to a city for a specific event, they impact the economy both inside and outside the sports arena.

Photo reprinted by permission of Jackie Kurkowski.

Demonstrating Value of Event or Operations

Some sport operations can attract visitors who spend money at their establishments. Increased business activity due to sport often results in the creation of new jobs. Yet, some local public officials may be oblivious to the size and extent of the economic impact created by the sport industry. Economic impact studies attempt to measure what a designated economy would be missing had an event or operation not occurred. By demonstrating the economic gain resulting from an attraction to various publics (e. g., government, residents, investors, media), greater support in the form of human and/or financial resources may be received in the future. Residents and government officials recognize the economic importance of the Green Bay Packers to their city. The economic impact of the preseason training camp alone is estimated to be $4 million annually.

fying the geographic origin and ultimate destination of expenditures.

Sport Tourism Economic Benefits

A continuum of economic benefits and costs exists for communities that host sport tourism events. These benefits include expenditures by sport tourists that, in turn, create local employment, personal income, and subsequent re-spending within an economy. Accompanying these transactions are tax dollars to governmental units and subsequent tax relief to residents within the jurisdiction of the taxing body. Sport tourism events may also internalize local income, inducing spending by residents at the expense of outside attractions. Economic cost impacts of sport tourism events include price inflation for tourism goods and services, opportunity, and substitution costs. Increases in crime, environmental degradation, and disruption of residents' lifestyles and patterns may also yield economic costs. Quantifying some of these impacts into economic terms is difficult, and that difficulty may be one reason why they are typically ignored.

Importance of Economic Impact Research in Sport

There are several reasons why economic impact studies are so popular in the world of sport. Each will be discussed in this section.

An economic impact study indicates that the inaugural Brickyard 400 NASCAR stock car race in 1996 had a direct impact of $31.5 million and a total impact of $60 million on the Indianapolis community. The analysis was limited to spending by tourists who were in Indianapolis specifically for the race. Spending of Indianapolis residents and non-residents who came to the city for business or personal reasons was not included. The first Brickyard 400, run without an infield crowd, attracted an estimated 310,000.

Findings from economic impact assessments, which include return on investment (ROI), need to be brought to the attention of sport managers and, more important, to budget decision-makers in local governments. Such data are meaningful and effective when demonstrating the contributions sport services make to a local community. Once aware of the potential economic benefits, local tourism industry managers also may be more inclined to support sport services in order to stimulate visitation during off-peak periods (seasonality).

Assisting in Attracting Sponsorships

Armed with information from an economic impact study, the sport marketer may confidently approach a prospective sponsor and describe the direct economic benefits sponsors may derive from their affiliation. Valid economic impact and market data generated can also assist the event organization in attracting sponsors, and such information should be included in event sponsor packages. Survey instruments should request spending behavior by service sector (i.e., lodging, retail spending, transportation, etc.). In the case of the Illinois High School Association (IHSA) Girls State Basketball Tournament, spectators spent over $500,000 for lodging during the weekend of the play-offs. This information is of particular value when seeking an exclusive sponsorship arrangement from a lodging provider (e.g., "Official" hotel of the 1995 IHSA State Basketball Championships).

The utility of any evaluation model is in its ability to generate valid for decision-making. In this regard, information derived from economic impact studies can assist sport marketers in their planning efforts. Inflated, inaccurate economic impact studies mislead publics and serve to discredit economic impact studies, in general.

Generating Consumer Market Profile

Information generated from an economic impact study has particular value in tracking the geographic origin of visitor groups and determining their expenditures at the attraction and elsewhere within the designated economy under study. The effectiveness of the attraction's promotional messages and images on selected geographic markets may also be ascertained. In this regard, the economic impact model may be extended to the degree to which promotional materials influenced visitors to attend an attraction or make additional purchases within the designated economy.

Even without a guarantee of an Olympic Games, Utah committed $59 million in state funds in 1989 to winter sports. It is estimated that Olympic visitors will spend $173 million and that Games-related jobs should generate up to half a billion dollars from 1997 to 2002.

Enhancing Organization's Image and Employee Morale

Positive results from an economic impact study may benefit the sport organization in qualitative ways. Richardson, Long, and Perdue (1989) found that employee morale and department status were elevated by results of economic evaluations.

Assisting Community Development Planning Process

Helping to Gain Public Sector Support for Sport Tourism Operations

Significant tax revenues may accrue to national, state/provincial, and local governments in locations where large-scale sporting events are held. Economic impact studies should attempt to measure the tax revenues attributed to the attraction and returned to various levels of government. Such findings may be of particular use to attraction marketers as "bargaining tools" when seeking financial support for their activities or service cost discounts from governmental units. Claiming that the expenditures would revitalize its urban environment, Atlanta invested $2.580 billion on the 1996 Summer Olympics, including $232 million on the new stadium and $194 million on the athletes' village.

Tow (1994) reported that local government units in New Zealand annually invest NZ$300 million in sport and leisure. Their return on investment is considerable, with sport and leisure spending contributing NZ$1.6 billion to the economy and supporting 23,000 full-time jobs.

Economic contributions of sporting events to the host community, over time, may attract new tourism-driven businesses or result in the expansion of existing businesses. Walt Disney World in Orlando, Florida, understands the economic stimulus sport tourism can create. In 1995, Disney broke ground on an 80-acre sport complex to host championship events, many in conjunction with the Amateur Athletic Union (AAU). Disney and the AAU have teamed to ensure that, by the year 2000, 40 national youth sport championships will be held at the newly constructed, $200-million sport complex. Disney's sport community features a 7,500-seat ballpark plus a baseball quadraplex, a fieldhouse that can accommodate 5,000 in an arena around a pro-sized hardwood court, a 12-court tennis center, a softball quadraplex, beach volleyball courts, four multipurpose playing fields sized for international soccer, and a track-and-field stadium (Turco & Eisenhardt, 1998).

Relatively smaller sporting events are attractive to smaller communities for their potential economic impacts. The 1999 International Tug of War attracted 2,500 competitors to Rochester, Minnesota. The National Trampoline and Tumbling games drew 4,000 to Ames, Iowa. Civic leaders estimated that each visitor spent about $120 a day at hotels, restaurants and stores. The World Horseshoe Tournament drew 1,300 pitchers to Eau Claire, Wisconsin. The 1999 Senior Open at Des Moines Golf and Country Club drew 252,800 fans for the weeklong event, and broke concession and merchandise sales records. Officials estimated tournament spectators would spend between $20–$25 million on meals, lodging, car rentals, etc. Iowa State University researchers estimated the economic impact, direct and indirect, as high as $60 million. Events at the Rockford, Illinois 100-acre sports facility featuring 10 soccer fields and eight championship softball fields, account for more than 60,000 hotel room bookings a year. With the stakes so high, increasingly, rights holders are bidding out their events to host communities. More competition among communities has created a seller's market in sport event bidding.

In the last 15 years, Indianapolis has realized significant financial returns on its $124-million amateur sport investment. Between 1977 and 1991, spending by out-of-town visitors attracted to Indianapolis by amateur sports totaled $787 million. Expenditures by sport organizations and facilities from external sources brought $213 and $51 million respectively to the Indianapolis economy. Indianapolis claims that the 1987 Pan American Games generated over $141 million in direct spending.

Economic Costs in Sport

Many sport economic impact studies have measured only economic benefits, excluding production and indirect costs. Sport economic impact analyses must be extended to include the costs as well as benefits. Such research becomes similar to cost-benefit analysis. Financial costs to produce a sporting event often include payment to local government units for such services as traffic control (police department), emergency medical rescue (fire department), and refuse collection (public works department), costs that account for as much as 40% of the operating budget (Turco, 1995). Income leakages from an economy via no-resident-allied event businesses, and increased prices to local residents in retail and restaurant establishments are other examples of economic costs associated with large-scale sport operations. Opportunity costs or changes in expenditure patterns may be attributed to people's staying away because of the perception that the sporting event would have inflated prices, crowds, and difficulties in finding accommodations. Zipp (1996) analyzed the degree to which the absence of baseball affected retail trade and hotel room sales in the 24 U.S. cities hosting baseball franchises and in 4 control cities. It was concluded that the strike had little, if any, economic impact on host cities. Retail trade appeared to be almost completely unaffected by the strike, and the declines in hotel room sales in 10 baseball cities were not consistent with decreases expected by changes associated with the strike.

Negative social-cost impacts of sport may include traffic congestion, vandalism, additional police and fire protection, environmental degradation, and disruption of residents' lifestyles and patterns. Quantifying some of these impacts into economic terms is difficult and may be one reason why they are typically ignored.

Steps to Conduct Economic Impact Research

Researchers have used a variety of data collection approaches and analyses, including recall surveys, expenditure diaries, and tax records, to assess the economic impacts of sport tourism. Often, the economic impact methodology is "tailored" to the specifics of a sport. The nature and location of the sport service to be studied, time, human and financial resources available will typically dictate the appropriate data collection methods. This section identifies the various steps and methods used to determine the economic impact of sporting events.

Step 1. Determine Scope of Study

The first step in sport economic impact assessment requires determining the scope of the study. This involves designating sources of economic impact, defining the local economy, and determining the types of information sought.

As with any form of field survey research, the type of information desired and the nature of the event dictate the scope of the study. Typically, nonresident participants and spectators are the primary sources of economic impact associated with sporting events and operations. An economic-impact researcher must decide which spending sources to include in the study. Obviously, the wider the scope of the study (more spending sources) and the larger the designated economy, the greater will be the economic impacts. Similarly, the more spending sources included, the more time and research resource requirements will be needed. It must be decided which sources of economic impact will be evaluated. Depending on the nature of the service, the following sources of economic impact may be studied: Participants, spectators, event-sponsoring organization, allied event businesses (e.g., souvenir vendors, food and beverage vendors, entertainers).

Again, depending on the scope of the study and on the nature and scale of the service, an economic impact study can be a large undertaking. The sport marketer must be realistic about the number of resources required to conduct an economic impact study. Does the sport organization have the staff expertise and availability to conduct such a study, or will an external consultant be required? Time, access of secondary information, and human and financial resources must be considered during this initial planning stage.

Sources of Economic Impact at Sport Tourism Events

Nonresident: a. Participants

           b. Spectators

           c. Event Organization

           d. Allied Businesses

               1. Food & Beverage Vendors

               2. Souvenir Vendors

               3. Exhibitors

               4. Entertainers

               5. Other (e.g. local retail outlets, gasoline stations, etc.)

Local economy

The affected geographic area or local economy must also be defined for proper economic impact analysis. Crompton (1995) lists this oversight as one of 11 methodological errors associated with sport economic impact research. Sporting events come in various shapes and sizes and may impact regional, metropolitan, county, city, or neighborhood economies. County and city economic areas are the preferred local economies for study because of the availability of financial records (i.e., sales and tax receipts) as well as their political boundaries. Examples of economies defined for previous studies are listed in Table 3.1.

Table 3.1. Examples of Designated Economies of Impact in Sport Tourism

Study	Local Economy
Kodak Albuquerque International Balloon Fiesta	Greater Albuquerque, NM
Oldsmobile Balloon Classic	Vermillion County, IL
1994 IHSA Girl's State Basketball Tournament	McLean County, IL
1996 Little Illini Soccer Fall Classic	Champaign-Urbana, IL
ASA Softball Tournament	McLean County, IL

Information requirements.

The type of information desired by the researcher will also dictate the scope of the economic impact assessment. An economic impact study of the 1993 Albuquerque International Balloon Fiesta provided organizers with spectator market profiles, spectator satisfaction levels, and financial return on investment information in addition to the event's direct economic impact.

Step 2. Select Data Collection Strategy

Once the scope of the economic impact study has been determined, a strategy must be developed that will yield valid and reliable data. Primary data collection techniques can be accurate and effective methods to determine sport spectator spending behaviors (Ritchie & Aitken, 1984). Large-scale sport events present several methodological challenges for researchers using primary data for impact analysis, as such events are typically held over several days, involve multiple events and venues, and attract large spectator crowds. Multiple entrance/exit points, concurrent event schedules, uncertainty of sport competitions, and in some cases, climatic conditions further compound the challenges. Most research on mega-sport events has involved field surveys of spectators and/or participants. Field survey research has been previously conducted on such diverse events as the Olympic Games (Ritchie & Aitken, 1984), Grand Prix automobile races (Burns & Mules, 1989), and hot air balloon championships (Turco, 1997) with the objectives to determine spectator market characteristics, event economic impacts, resident attitudes, and event promotional effectiveness.

There are numerous data collection techniques that have been employed in economic impact research studies, each with advantages and disadvantages. This section provides an overview of field survey approaches used for economic impact analysis of sport events and describes several accompanying methodological issues associated with sampling and data collection. It is up to the economic impact researcher and the agency commissioning the study to select the method or methods most appropriate for their event.

Less labor-intensive ways of estimating sport tourism economic impacts often involve analyzing local business receipts, tax rolls, and/or other sources of secondary data. If there has been no change in the economy under study, other than the injection of dollars attributed to the sport service, use of these secondary data sources is appropriate to determine economic impact. The difficulty in using business receipts and tax records for economic impact studies centers on attribution. Is the change in the sales due to the sport service or to some other occurrence? Further, private sector business records might not be readily accessible, as owners are often reluctant to share their information with "outsiders." State and local tax records are usually released quarterly, adding a time delay to economic impact calculations.

Survey questions for economic impact assessment. If primary data are to be collected from surveys, at least the questions featured in Figure 3.2 should be posed. Categories of on-site spending vary, depending on the nature of the event, and may include food and beverages, souvenirs, and entertainment; off-site expenditure categories often request expenditure information on lodging, meals, retail shopping, gasoline, and miscellaneous purchases.

Where do you live? City   State   Zip Code   Country

How many nonresidents are in your visitor group?

How much will your nonresident group members spend on the event grounds this trip?

       Amusements/Entertainment _____   Food/Beverage _____

       Gifts/Souvenirs _____   Other _____

How much will your nonresident group members spend in *(name of local economy)* this trip?

       Lodging _____   Meals _____

       Retail Shopping _____   Other _____

Optional Questions

How many times will your group attend *(name of the event)* this trip? _____

Had the *(name of the event)* not been held, would you have visited another community outside of the *(name of local economy)* area today? 1. ____ yes   2. ____ no   3. ____ not sure

a. If yes, what would have been the length of your stay outside of *(name of local economy)*? _____night

---

Figure 3.2. Essential Economic Impact Survey Questions

Summary. Researchers have used various survey data collection techniques to estimate the economic impact of sport, including diaries, on-site interviews, and mail-back surveys, each with advantages and disadvantages. The advantages of on-site interviews are that interviewer may interpret questions that may at first be difficult for the tourist to understand and the data are retained by the researcher and not subject to time delays, as may be the case with mail-back surveys or expenditure diaries. A disadvantage with the interview process is financial cost for interviewers, particularly for sport tourism experiences that are seasonal or events that are several days in duration. Mail-back surveys are less labor intensive for the researcher but are subject to low response rates. Further, as more time passes from the point of tourism experience to the survey, there is greater likelihood that the respondents will underestimate their spending.

The future of field survey research in sport will include voice-activated, hand-held microcomputers linked to cellular phone lines for instant collection and analysis. Research methods should be tailored to the specifics of the event and not be standardized. The nature and duration of the sport event, the time it takes for data collection, and the human and financial resources of the research organization dictate the most practical data collection methods. However, care must be taken to design and implement survey research methods that will negate the aforementioned contaminants to validity.

Step 3. Compute Direct Economic Impact.

The next step in determining the economic impacts of a sport tourism event involves the calculation of direct spending. The worksheets on the national bicycling championships that follow were prepared to help determine the sport spectator and participant spending. Before calculating the event's economic impact, the following information is required:

- Event spectator attendance totals

- Number of other nonresident visitors (day trippers)

- Estimation of total overnight visitors

- Estimation of repeat spectators (if event is more than 1 day in duration)

- Average direct spending by participants and/or spectators by selected expenditure categories.

The above information may be obtained from field surveys at the event. The example involving the National Bicycling Championships is provided on the following pages to illustrate the calculations necessary to determine the impacts of sport on a designated economy.

Example—National Bicycling Championships:

Event spectator attendance:. 10,000

Total overnight visitors (13%). 1,300

Other nonresident visitors (21% day trippers). 2,100

Table 3.2 reveals per person, per day spending estimates of spectators. Note: Average direct spending figures and information on spectator length of stay are derived from a spectator survey.

Table 3.2

Number of nonresident spectators		
Day trippers: _____ × $ _____ direct spending = $ _____		
Overnight guests: _____ × _____ nights × $ _____ direct spending = $ _____		
Spectator Example: National Bicycling Championships		
Day trippers:	2,100 × $23 avg. direct spending =	$48,300
Overnight guests:	1,300 × 2 nights × $110 avg. direct spending =	$286,000
Total spectator direct impact:		$ 334,300

Table 3.3 reveals per person, per day spending estimates of participants. Note: Average participant length of stay and their direct spending figures are derived from a participant survey.

It is acceptable to include the local spending of the event-producing organization in the total direct economic impact calculation. (Please see Table 3.3.)

Table 3.3

Number of nonresident participants/teams		
Day trippers: _____ × $ _____ direct spending = $ _____		
Overnight guests: _____ × _____ nights × $ _____ direct spending = $ _____		
Participant Example: National Bicycling Championships		
Day trippers:	145 × $48 average direct spending =	$ 6,960
Overnight guests:	210 × 3 nights × $164 direct spending =	$103,320
Total participant direct impact:		$110,280

Table 3.4. Direct Economic Impact of the National Bicycling Championships

Event organization—local spending	$38,201
Total spectator direct impact	334,300
Total participant direct impact	110,280
Total	**$482,781**

Economic Impact Calculations

Another worksheet useful in computing the direct economic impacts of sport tourism events is provided below:

1. Total Event or Service Attendance	_____
2. Percent Nonresidents (NR)	_____
3. NR Attendance (Multiply 1 by 2)	_____
4. Average Visitor Group Size	_____
5. NR Visitor Groups (Divide 3 by 4)	_____
6. Average Spending by NR Groups	_____
7. Total Spending by NR Groups	_____
(Multiply 5 by 7)	_____

Example:

1. Total Event or Service Attendance	50,000
2. Percent Nonresidents (NR)	× .250
3. NR Attendance (Multiply 1 by 2)	12,500
4. Average Visitor Group Size	÷ 2.2
5. NR Visitor Groups (Divide 3 by 4)	5,682
6. Average Spending by NR Groups	× $107.47
7. Total Spending by NR Groups	

Econometric Models

Several statistical models have been used to estimate the economic impacts of tourism. The *input-output* (IO) model permits the calculation of aggregate multiplier coefficients for different sectors of an economy, such as food and drink, lodging, and entertainment, and demonstrates the interrelationships between different sectors at a given time. The United States Department of Agriculture (USDA) Forest Service IMPLAN (Impact Analysis for PLANning) system contains input-output models for all states and counties in the United States and has been widely adopted as the regional impact analysis program of choice. An alternative is the RIMS and RIMS II (Regional Input-Output Modeling System) developed by the U.S. Department of Commerce Bureau of Economic Analysis, which also offers input-output tables at the county level. Gazel and Schwer (1997) discuss the strengths and weaknesses of IO models:

A comparison of three IO models (REMI-II, IMPLAN, and REMI) conducted by Rickman and Schwer (1995) found no significant difference in multipliers after benchmarking the models, although the models differ substantially. They conclude that the "ready-to-use" IO-based models offer an appropriate format for conducting the indirect effects as part of an economic impact study.

A major criticism of IO models is the use of fixed coefficient (Leontieff-type) production functions that assume no substitution between the different production factors. For most staged tourism events this assumption is not a problem since the economic impacts are short-term which are consistent with a fixed technology. A more significant problem is that most regional IO models are comprised by regionalizing national coefficients. The relative low cost make IO models attractive for use in economic impact studies.

Issues in Economic Impact Research

Crompton (1995) described several contributors to inaccurate economic impact analysis, including use of sales multipliers instead of household income multipliers. Failure to accurately identify the impacted area, failure to exclude "time-switchers" and "casuals," omission of opportunity costs, measurement of only benefits while omitting costs, and inclusion of local spectators.

We will cover the issue of multipliers later in the chapter and have already discussed the importance of accurately designating economies for impact analysis. Crompton (1995) advises that expenditures from time-switchers and casuals be factored out of economic impact computations. He describes these two segments of the event visitor market as follows:

Some nonlocal spectators at a sports event may have been planning a visit to the community for a long time but changed the timing of their visit to coincide with the event. Their spending cannot be attributed to the vent, because it would have been made without the event, albeit at a different time of the year. Other visitors may have already been in the community, attracted by other features, and may have elected to go to the sports event instead of doing something else. (p. 27)

Most economic impact researchers have avoided calculating resident spending associated with sport tourism attractions. They have surmised that in the short run, spending by local sports fans may not represent a net increase in economic activity, but is merely a diversion of leisure dollars from other activities within an economy. Researchers argue that people have only so much to spend on entertainment. Spending at home games comes out of personal income that otherwise might go for movie or theater tickets, concerts, museums, or theme parks. However, it is appropriate to include local spending if it would have been taken outside the economy had not the port team been playing. The question then is how to determine what locals might have been spent elsewhere.

Recently, some researchers have correctly identified another economic impact variable, spending by local area residents within the economy that would not have occurred locally in the absence of the event in question. This effect, termed *income substitution*, may be a significant component of total economic impact. Cobb and Weinberg (1993) concluded that import substitution effects are comparable to those produced from exports (spending by nonlocals in the local economy). They believe that ignoring import substitution effect may significantly underestimate the true incremental impact of local events. Some local events tend to draw more heavily than others from the local population.

Negative or cost impacts of tourism events and attractions may include traffic congestion, vandalism, additional police and fire protection, environmental degradation, increased prices to local residents in retail and eating and drinking establishments, and disruption of residents' lifestyles and patterns.

Multipliers

A local economy comprises many businesses that buy from and sell to other businesses within the area and outside the region. Multiplier coefficients take into account the interrelationships of businesses within a designated economy. The more independent or self-sufficient the economy, the greater will be the multiplier coefficient.

The basic idea of the multiplier is that direct tourist spending in an area does not stop as soon as the dollars have been spent. A portion of tourist spending re-circulates through the local economy before leaking out to pay for basic purchases elsewhere. The portion of re-spending that stays in the economy is the multiplier effect, and that portion that is lost to economies where goods and services were purchased and imported, is termed *leakage*.

When using multiplier coefficients for impact analysis, it is necessary that they correspond to the geographic area under study. Multiplier co-efficients will be higher where a greater proportion of spending is in sectors with strong links to other industries and businesses. Lodges, shops, and other services are examples of businesses directly supported by visitor spending. Only nonresident attraction visitors create a net stimulus to the designated economy. Even though residents of the local area may spend money at or near the tourism attraction, presumably they would have spent that money in the economy on other goods and services. It is, therefore, inappropriate to apply multiplier coefficients to expenditures made by local residents in their home area.

Generally, the greater the geographic area, the larger will be the multiplier. Larger geographic areas will contain wholesale and retail tourism suppliers from which local businesses may purchase goods and services (inputs). The U.S. Department of Commerce Travel and Tourism Division reported output multiplier coefficients for 90% of all counties in the United States range from 1.40 to 1.80. Because multiplier coefficients for a single county are typically smaller than coefficients for a region comprising several counties, regional input-output multiplier coefficients may not be appropriate for economic impact studies involving attractions in rural communities.

Several types of multiplier coefficients are used in sport tourism impact assessments. *Sales multipliers* measure direct, indirect, and induced effects of an extra unit of visitor spending on economic activity within a community. This may not be as useful as income and employment multipliers because it is not only the volume of visitor sales that is important but also the portion of expenditures that ends up as local income. *Income multipliers* measure direct, indirect, and induced effects of an extra unit of visitor spending on the change in level of household income incomes in the economy. *Employment multipliers* measure direct, indirect, and induced effects of an extra unit of visitor spending on employment in the economy. This type of multiplier reveals the number of full-time equivalent (FTE) job opportunities supported by visitor expenditures.

As money is spent in an economy, it changes hands several times. To measure the multiplier effect, attention must be placed on how much total business or income results from the initial transaction. The individuals and businesses receiving payment return a portion of it to the income stream in the form of payment for expenses. The portion of spending returned outside the designated economy is termed leakage and no longer creates business activity or income within the economy. The portions of the initial transaction retained within the economy determine the true multiplier.

Individuals create leakage as they save a portion of income before spending the remainder. They may also spend some outside the economy on vacations, mail-order purchases, federal taxes, and other such activities. The businessperson has expenses that result in leakages—suppliers of goods and services may be out of the economy. As suppliers are paid, the money tends to move out of the economy.

To calculate the total economic impact of an original transaction, the amounts returned each time to the income stream are added until the return reaches zero. Figure 3.3 illustrates this process, depicting value added, turnover, and a multiplier. The value added is found in the breakdown of the original dollar expenditure. The dollar represents expenditure for the acquisition of goods and services. Value added is the change in value ($.85 occurring within the designated economy before the first turnover). The first turnover results in $.60 going outside the economy, representing federal taxes and other purchases. The remaining $.40 is the portion retained within the economy for wages, salaries, local taxes, rent, etc. Subsequent turnovers represent similar transactions as some money leaves and some remains.

The multiplier is the original dollar purchase and that part of the dollar that remains within the state on the various turnovers: First $1.00, then $.40, then $.15, then $.06, then $.02, then $.01 remains. At this point it becomes difficult to measure further impacts of the initial transaction.

The standard formula for a general income multiplier for an economy in which new income is introduced is as follows:

$$\text{income multiplier} = \frac{1}{1 - (x)\,(y)\,(z)}$$

Where x = percentage of the new income a consumer will spend rather than save;

y = percentage of consumer expenditure made in the economy under study; and,

z = percentage of business expenditure made in the economy under study.

To illustrate, assume that a person spends 90% of his total income, and 80% of that is spent within a designated economy. The business person from whom this individual buys goods and services must obtain most goods and services (60%) from outside the economy, retaining in the economy 40% of what the consumer initially spent. Taking these estimates:

$$1.4 \text{ income multiplier} = \frac{1}{1 - (.80)\,(.90)\,(.40)}$$

If $100 of new income were introduced to an economy, the final economic impact would be $140, which includes the original $100.

Sport Tourist Spending Patterns

How much does the average sport tourist spend per trip/night? It depends on the nature of the sporting event and characteristics of the host economy. Some sports attract high-end consumer groups (e.g., downhill skiing, golf, ballooning, yachting). One would surmise that per capita visitor spending would be higher among spectators and participants who attend such upscale events. However, one must be careful of such generalizations as certain sporting events not noted for attracting affluent markets also generate considerable net impacts on a local economy. For example, the World Horseshoe Tournament drew 1,300 pitchers to Eau Claire, Wisconsin and generated an estimated $1.4 million in spending for lodging, meals, and retail shopping. The National Trampoline and Tumbling Games attracted 4,000 to Ames, Iowa. Civic leaders estimated that each visitor spent an average of $120 per day on hotel stays, eating, drinking, and souvenirs.

As revealed on the next page, different sports stimulate different tourist spending behaviors. Typically, youth sporting events impact an economy more than those for young adults, because youths are often accompanied by parents or guardians, thereby attracting a larger visitor group (Turco, 1997).

Sport contests for older adults (e.g., Senior Olympics) and people with disabilities (e.g., Paralympics, Special Olympics) that attract significant numbers of nonresident participants and spectators are also desirable for some communities as participants and spectators may stay longer and be accompanied by more companions than are younger participants and those without disabilities. Players and fans attending the 1994 Senior Softball World Series in Orlando rented 4,907 rooms for at least one night, generating an estimated economic impact of $1.8 million (Mitchell, 1995).

The spatial proximity/distance of participating teams in relationship to the host economy also influences the economic impacts of sport tourism events. Teams within or adjacent to the host economy typically attract residents as spectators and generate fewer net dollars. In contrast, teams from greater distances often stay overnight in the host community and stimulate spectators to do the same within the host economy, thereby generating more impact. As the geographic origins of tournament teams changes from year to year, so too will their economic impacts on the host economy.

The prestige of an event as perceived by the sport tourist also influences the size of the visitor group and its spending. The Little League World Series is a once-in-a-lifetime opportunity for most participants, often

Sport Tourism Event Spending Profiles

Illinois High School Association Girls State Basketball Championship, Normal, Illinois

Scope of study: Direct, tax impacts
Spending sources: Spectator groups
Research methods: On-site, self-administered survey with incentive to complete
Spending profiles: Overnighters: $427.23/group (Avg. 4 persons/group)

Gus Macker 3-on-3 Basketball Tournament, Champaign-Urbana, Illinois

Scope of study: Direct, tax impacts
Spending sources: Player, spectator groups
Research methods: Mail-back survey to nonresident players
Spending profiles: Daytrippers: $139.12/group (Avg. 5 persons/group)
Overnighters: *$197.72/group (Avg. 4 persons/group)*

American Softball Association Men's National Championship, Bloomington, Illinois

Scope of study: Direct, tax, return on investment (ROI)
Spending sources: Teams, organization, spectators
Research methods: Spectators—On-site survey
Players—Mail-back survey to team managers
Organization—Event balance sheet
Spending profiles: Teams*: $4,403.40/team*
Organization: $121,876.00
Spectators: $316.56/group (Avg. 2 *persons/group*)

Family Circle Professional Women's Tennis Tournament, Hilton Head Island, South Carolina

Scope of study: Direct, indirect, total, tax impacts
Spending sources: Spectators
Research methods: On-site interviews
Spending profiles: Locals: $122.61/person
Overnighters: *$182.84/person*

attracting large numbers of spectators who are relatives/friends of the participants. It had been 30 years since the Green Bay Packers of the National Football League (NFL) had participated in the Super Bowl before their appearance in 1997. The novelty of their appearance in the title game triggered an unparalleled level of spending among Packer fans. In 1998, the team returned to the Super Bowl. Sales of Super Bowl XXXI merchandise, most of it featuring the Green Bay Packers, hit a record-setting $130 million.

The perceived attractiveness of the host community (i.e., alternative attractions, climate, proximity to relatives, friends, etc.) also may elicit larger visitor groups and stimulate relatively more spending from tourists. This is one of the reasons that Walt Disney World executives decided to venture further into the world of sport.

Sport Tour: It Pays to Play

A recent study suggests that hosting youth sporting events may make dollars and cents for a community. The annual Little Illini Orange & Blue Soccer Tournament held in Champaign-Urbana comprises over 100 boys' and girls' teams from eight states. Teams invited to participate in the tournament were at the top of their state's youth soccer rankings. In 1996, the weekend event attracted 1,725 nonresident participants and 2,500 parents/coaches/chaperons. The tournament was held in the "twin" cities of Champaign and Urbana, Illinois, located approximately 110 miles south of Chicago. Champaign County was used as the designated economy for study.

An expenditure questionnaire was included in the registration packets of all nonresident players. Registration packets were given to the participants' parents/guardians (N=791) upon check-in. In the accompanying cover letter, parents/guardians were instructed to complete the postage-paid, return-addressed questionnaire within one month of the tournament. A drawing for a $100 U.S. Savings Bond was used as an incentive to complete the survey. A total of 120 questionnaires, representing 420 individuals, were returned and deemed usable for analysis.

Expenditure data were requested at the visitor group level rather than by individuals. The analysis for this study was limited to direct economic impacts, excluding sales or income multipliers.

Results of a survey revealed that tournament visitor groups spent, on average, $294.09 in the local economy, primarily on lodging (39.2%), meals (30.2%), and retail shopping (13.7%). Visitors spent an average of $55.76 per person, per day in local economy. The event generated $376,077 in direct expenditures and $8,957 in local tax revenues, of which $6,844 was from lodging. Was the event a good deal economically for the host community? Considering the cash outlay for the city to host the event was $7,240, it appears the tournament generated a small return on investment.

1. Define the following terms: economic impact, multiplier, leakage, import substitution, expenditure switching.

Discussion Questions

2. Identify an economy that is influenced by sport as a focal attraction. Describe the businesses most influenced by the sport attraction and their spatial relationships to the sport site(s).

3. Compare and contrast the advantages and disadvantages of the different data collection techniques used to assess the economic impacts of sport tourism.

Chapter 4

Designing Sport Tourism Events

Questions

1. *What is the process for conducting a feasibility study of a sport tourism event?*
2. *What planning steps are necessary for bidding to host a sport tourism event?*
3. *What are the stages of the sport tourism event strategic planning process?*

Introduction

Sport tourism events are globally significant in terms of their ability to generate popular appeal and their use as a strategy used by communities to attract investment. This chapter focuses on key considerations to stage successful sport tourism events and additional factors that need to be examined in the future are highlighted. First, sport tourism events are defined, and the initial phases of designing a sport tourism event are considered. They include research, and emphasis is placed on both an informal assessment and formal appraisal of the event under consideration. The importance of undertaking a feasibility study and understanding the event bidding process is highlighted. The event planning process is a lengthy one, and careful attention to a number of critical planning aspects is warranted. It includes consideration of the market plan, the business plan, and the strategic plan of the event. Other factors requiring consideration, such as organizational structure, timeline, setting and location considerations, are further described. Finally, attention to factors causing unsuccessful events and future considerations for communities planning to host sport tourism events are highlighted. Although this chapter emphasizes basic considerations that can be applied to the designing of successful events, in general, it is imperative that the event organizer recognize the uniqueness of the event in order to identify the differences and the associated implications.

As previously noted, sport tourism events comprise those events in which the primary purpose for travel is participating in or viewing of sport. It is important to note that sport tourism events are extremely diverse. A sports-for-all festival, the X-Games, a youth soccer tournament, a Masters long course swimming championship, and a ultra-marathon race are all examples of sport tourism events. Therefore, every event should be regarded as different, and to ignore their uniqueness can lead to poor organization that could easily be avoided.

Definition of Sport Tourism Events

Goldblatt (1997) contends that the better research one conducts prior to the proposed event, the greater the probability that one will produce an event that matches the planned outcomes of the organization. Moreover, it is necessary for event organizers to spend more time on researching and evaluating events. In order to reduce the risk of nonattendance of an event, it is essential to conduct an informal assessment as well as a formal appraisal of the need to host an event.

Importance of Research

The increasing proliferation of events worldwide has sparked a desire by many communities to host an event without meticulous consideration of the consequences. Before commencing on hosting an event, it is imperative to answer a number of questions concerning the endeavor. Why a community needs or wants to hold an event is probably the most important question of all (Watt, 1992). Cities and nations host events for a number of reasons. For example, one of the primary objectives for the Cape Town Olympic bid was that it would be developmental. In other words, the hosting of the Games would be placed at the service of development as the plan was to provide sport facilities in the deprived communities. The Barbados Government emphasizes the hosting of sport tourism events in order to further the development of sport, while simultaneously promoting Barbados as an international sporting destination. Often, there must be a series of compelling motivations that justify the significance and viability of hosting the event.

Informal Assessment of the Need to Host an Event

Once a city or region knows why it would like to host an event, it is essential to know the nature of the event: What is the event product? The event could be an annual 10km run or a sports festival comprising a number of events. Some events may require the submission of an actual bid document. This issue will be discussed in greater depth later. It is also important to consider when the event will take place. Clashes with other events in the city or region can be disastrous. At this stage, it would be a good idea to consult such media representatives as TV broadcasters. They will be able to advise when the most appropriate times for an event will be so that it does not clash with other, maybe more important, events. For example, when Cape Town chose the dates for the hosting of the 2004 Olympic, they were informed that it would clash with the World Series baseball coverage. "When" may also determine where the event will be held.

A crucial factor in determining an event's success is the geographical location. Where the event will take place (i.e., city, state, or country) as well as the venue (i.e., stadium, golf course, beachfront) needs to be considered. Convenience to transport links and other amenities is key in determining an event's location. In other words, the host community and sport venue must be easily accessible.

Another critical factor that needs to be considered at this early stage of an event organization is funding. It may be regarded as perhaps one of the key items for hosting an event, and is covered thoroughly in Chapter 7. As competition for events intensifies and government funding is cut back, it is important to know that you will have the funding to proceed. It will in all probability be financially damaging for a city/region to embark on an event without the necessary financial guarantees in place.

Finally, it is necessary to consider how the event will be achieved and who is going to be involved in the organization of it. Consideration as to "who" will be the stakeholders of the event will help determine the level of commitment of each grouping and better define those for whom the event is being produced (Goldblatt, 1997). A specific audience will have to be targeted. Moreover, prospective opposition to the event should further be determined. The organization, Bread Not Circuses, that expressed opposition to the proposed hosting of the 1996 Olympic Games in Toronto exemplified such opposition. Whether the event occurs on a small scale or a large scale, it is important to ensure that an organizational structure and an achievable plan be put in place—they will differ only in terms of complexity. The relative simplicity of some events does not eliminate the need to think them through (Watt, 1992).

After one has considered all these questions and has a positive attitude toward embarking on an event, a more formal appraisal should be considered, especially if the event is of a significant size or cost.

Formal Appraisal of the Need to Host an Event

The formal appraisal stage can be considered as more detailed planning. If an event is to succeed, it has to do so as a result of planned action. An event does just happen. Watt (1992) notes that planning is the process that identifies aims and objectives, and establishes the methods to be utilized to achieve these objectives. The formal appraisal process starts with undertaking a feasibility study and specifying the aims and objectives of the event.

A feasibility study asks the same kind of questions posed earlier but in a more specific manner. It looks at viable methods of accomplishing the event and identifying possible sources of funding. Moreover, a feasibility study aims to gather research information concerning the community and special interests groups for use as a decision-making tool by the community (Farmer, Mulrooney, & Ammon., 1996). Similarly, Getz (1997) reports that a feasibility study often implies an assessment of affordability or profitability; however, it should also be viewed as a comprehensive evaluation of the desirability and suitability of an event proposal. Getz (1997) further notes that the study should play a role in the destination's tourism plan. The politics of attracting events is often bizarre; irrationality rather than sound planning tends to accompany the pursuit of events, particularly major sport tourism events.

An informal group of specialist consultants, depending on the level of the event, can be employed to give a detailed report. Schmader and Jackson (1997) suggest that in most cases, feasibility studies should be conducted by qualified professionals who can provide meaningful projections based on current knowledge and tend to be more objective than those involved in event planning and production. This report is often performed within a short timescale. Yet, as noted by Schmader and Jackson, a study can take from a few weeks to several months or even a year, particularly if a master plan is required upon completion of the study. For new and large events, especially, Schmader and Jackson recommend that these events not be presented until a year or more after the feasibility study. The feasibility study should confirm that the venue, host community, and destination area have the capability to absorb the event and its impacts (Getz, 1997). The feasibility study should show recommendations on the method of achievement if the event is to be justifiable.

Questions to Be Considered for a Feasibility Study

Feasibility studies consist of a number of questions that have to be carefully considered. Positive answers will lead to more detailed planning. The following questions may be used as a guide to assess the plausibility of embarking on an event.

Type of event. For those who do not have a specific event in mind, one should determine which event will be the best attraction and have the greatest prospect of success. The type of event can vary, depending on a number of factors such as geographic location, size and age of population, weather, ability of the organizers, and facilities and services available.

A number of factors that require careful analysis and weighting, such as the weather, competition, population and attitude, amongst others, will be further outlined.

Weather. Weather can strongly influence the timing and success of the event, even if the event is staged indoors. Inclement weather can keep the crowds away, and this will in all probability have a negative effect on media effort and on the ultimate success of the event. Without doubt, weather is a greater consideration for events staged outdoors. According to Schmader and Jackson (1997), research should assist in selecting a time when the specific area has a greater than 80% chance of having weather suitable to promote attendance and facilitate event presentation. Weather reports and information can be obtained from weather bureaus, airport meteorological stations, and universities. It is recommended that weather patterns over a significant period of time be analyzed.

Competition. Careful consideration and attention should be given to all events occurring around the proposed time of the event, even if the activities planned are not in direct competition. It is an important aspect to note because most events rely heavily on the media for publicity. Schmader and Jackson (1992) suggest that new events be scheduled so that they do not occur around the same period of more established events that will most likely receive more media attention.

Major national occasions should further be considered as they will have an effect on local attendance. For example, it would be very difficult to stage an event in on the day of the Currie Cup Rugby final in South Africa or Super Bowl Sunday in the United States.

As a result of heightened competition, small to midsize communities may be at an advantage for hosting sport tourism events. In these communities, the diverse groups and interests present in larger communities may not be as prevalent (Catherwood & Van Kirk, 1992). In addition, larger cities may have too many competing events that detract attention from the specific sport tourism event.

In view of the effect that competing events may have on the proposed period of an event, it is essential to consult resources such as event calendars, which will detail times of upcoming events. This information can also be obtained from local and national sporting bodies, tourism and convention bureaus, and the Internet.

Population. Demographic research is of vital importance to a feasibility study. It is necessary to establish whether there will be enough people interested in the proposed event. Schmader and Jackson (1997) contend that the number of people within the event marketing radius must first be determined. The event radius will vary, depending on whether it is a city or regional event. Moreover, factors such as average income, age strata, unemployment percentages, minority groupings, and predicted growth or decline patterns for these factors should further be considered (Schmader & Jackson, 1997). This information can be obtained from a census bureau and other governmental agencies. The national or local sport association may further provide information about the popularity of a sport in a particular region.

Attitudes. Although attitude may be considered a more subjective measure than some of the others presented here, it is important to ascertain how those targeted to participate or attend actually feel about the proposed event. Focus groups or personal interviews as opposed to questionnaires should be used as a measure of attitude. Schmader and Jackson (1997) contend that questionnaires rarely afford an opportunity to provide an adequate event description. Therefore, news media polls do not offer an effective gauge of public reaction to a proposed event.

More meaningful attitude profiles can be obtained through well-designed personal interview strategies. As interviews take up a considerable amount of time, it may be wise to consider hiring professionals to conduct such studies, especially if a major event is being considered. Interviewees should be selected from a wide range of private sector and community organizations, such as commerce and industry, cultural and financial pursuits, educational and civic groups, law enforcement and other governmental agencies. Representatives of organizations directly related to the theme of the event, such as the local, regional, and national sport bodies should also be interviewed.

Community support. This factor, although one of considerable importance, is often neglected. Getz (1997) notes that public input is essential at this stage to ascertain levels of support or opposition and to resolve issues. The community should not be asked merely to attend the event; they should be involved from the start. Local residents should, therefore, be involved in consultation and decision-making processes. They are a valuable source of input and should not be neglected. For world-class events, it is of vital importance to ensure that one has the backing of every necessary group. Getz (1997) recommends an open debate concerning the value of the proposed event and a political decision taken to proceed, or not. He adds that communities generally are not asked their opinion. The importance of community support is further underscored because residents have to put up with the negatives associated with an event (e.g., congestion, noise, use of their tax dollars). However, formal political approval through referendum or council vote is only necessary if public resources have to be committed.

Consideration should be given to whether local organizations support events in a meaningful manner and whether they are genuinely enthusiastic about hosting them. The importance of volunteer help from the community will contribute to the success of the event. One further has to consider whether the attendance figures are reasonable, irrespective of whether it is a free or paid event.

Government leaders are playing an increasingly important role in event oversight (Goldblatt, 1997). Politicians may view events as both positive (in terms of economic impact) or negative (drain on municipal services). Therefore, it is important to enlist the support of governmental agencies and politicians in order to facilitate event functioning.

Community reputation. Cities and regions that have a reputation for hosting successful events should, in all probability, have a better chance of hosting subsequent events. Moreover, reasonable accommodation, food, and merchandise price structure and low crime rates, are considered plus factors for a city submitting a proposal for an event. The omission of any of these properties necessitates consideration of how these factors can be corrected or controlled. For communities that have never hosted major sport tourism events, the key to attracting one is to first decide the event the community will support.

Facilities and services. Because an event usually centralizes large numbers of attendees in a compact space, it will be necessary to ensure that the space will be efficient and safe. Moreover, vehicular and pedestrian patterns need to be adequately controlled. For major events, public transportation may be required. Lack of convenient public transportation to various venues was a major criticism of the 1996 Summer Olympic Games in Atlanta. One further needs to ensure that there are adequate facilities to accommodate event needs such as venues, accommodations, and related services. Venue selection may be limited by the type of the event and the availability within the region (Graham, Goldblatt & Delpy, 1995). If additional facilities are required, it will be necessary to consider whether this demand can be met through construction of temporary facilities. Moreover, consideration needs to be given to personnel requirements. One is required to ensure the presence of sufficient personnel, with expertise and work specialties, to implement the event successfully.

Funding and sponsorships. Watt (1992) contends that the biggest and most common error in embarking on an event is not securing funding at an early stage. Similarly, Getz (1997) reports that many bids proceed on the basis that "if we commit ourselves, can we raise the money?"

Therefore, financial viability should be a key point of the feasibility study. In today's world, it is evident that corporate sponsorship plays a large and continually growing role in event revenue support. Public and private sector partnerships in the hosting of the event are increasing. Schmader and Jackson (1997) suggest that the feasibility study should pivot on the availability of sponsorship. The history of local firms who support events should be listed. The likelihood of their financial involvement in the planned event should further be reported. If the planned event is big enough to warrant national sponsorship, investigations into best candidates at this level is important to the feasibility study. Risk assessment is also vital at this stage (Getz, 1997). Factors such as what happens if the revenues fail to materialize and costs escalate should be considered.

Partnerships. As previously noted, a main aspect of event organization is partnerships. Partnerships are relationships between two or more organizations responsible for the planning and implementation of a sport tourism event. It is worthwhile to establish partnerships early in the planning phase so that all stakeholders are involved from the very beginning. Problems can be expected as stakeholders may bring different motives to the event; however, a partnership is required to allow for sufficient finance and resources to be made available for a successful event. It is, therefore, important to identify possible partners who can bring their special skills, resources, and funding to an event. Moreover, all stakeholders should identify what they expect to get out of the event.

Environmental impact assessment. A formal environmental impact assessment (EIA) might be necessary during the feasibility stage, or possibly after the decision to embark on the event is made (Getz, 1997). Getz (1997) further notes that EIA legislation varies among jurisdictions; however, they may share following elements:

1. Description of all actions likely to have environmental impacts (on land, water, and air resources; on the built environment; on social/cultural circumstances and ecological systems).

2. Determination or prediction of the possible kinds of impacts and related uncertainties and risks.

3. Determination or prediction of the probable direction (positive or negative) and severity of impacts.

4. Plans for avoiding and curtailing possible negative impacts, achieving positive impacts, and improving any consequent problems.

5. Evaluation of benefits and costs of the project in lieu of impact predictions and plans.

A "Yes" Feasibility Study	If the outcome of the feasibility is positive, it will reveal the most suitable event for the host community, or it will support the event in mind. Moreover, it will outline the way forward to achieving the event, detailing structures, personnel requirements, financial resources, and an event achievement timescale (Watt, 1992). This will allow more detailed event planning and implementation to proceed given that enough time is allowed. Schmader and Jackson (1997) recommend that the report be consulted regularly because it is often laid aside once the initial interest has declined.

Event Bidding Considerations	In most instances of considering to host an event, one will be required to convince the owner of the event that one has the capability of successfully conducting the event. To accomplish this, one will need to consider a bid submission. A bid or application to host an event is a series of procedures outlining the steps one intends to carry out and the services one plans to provide to successfully stage an event (Wilkinson, 1988). Moreover, Wilkinson points out that the actions must satisfy the requirements and conditions of the organization that controls the event.

The bid submission is the initial commitment one makes on behalf of the city or municipality to the organization that controls the event. By this process, the organization ascertains the resources and plans presented by the host community. In some cases, one may be required to obtain guarantees that one will adhere to certain rules and regulations that govern the event (Wilkinson, 1988).

Different sports have different bidding processes and different objectives when allocating an event. Some may argue that an event should be placed in a city in which the sport is popular to attract a large audience. However, many sport organizations attempt to diversify the sites of their championship events in order to expand the scope of their sport. The National Collegiate Athletic Association (NCAA) water polo committee considered this an important factor despite the fact that 90% of the elite athletes are from California (Terrazas, 1995). Many international sporting bodies are favoring bids in South Africa in order to establish a base for their sport in other parts of the world. Cape Town won the right to host the World Senior Fencing Championships and the World Junior Cycling Championships and the World Junior Weightlifting Championships in 1997.

Some sports operate on a rotation basis, such as United States Swimming (USS; Terrazas, 1995). Terrazas indicates that USS is favoring bids from southern regions for the 1997 junior national meet provided they meet the criteria set out by the USS. The bid process consists of both a written agreement and an oral presentation to verify what the written bid submission disclosed. The written agreement for many sport tourism events entails responding to a Request for Proposal (RFP; Catherwood & Van Kirk, 1992). RFPs consist of documents in which the governing body specifies the guidelines and procedures for submitting a bid proposal. They usually include a specific list of questions to be answered by the bidding city concerning factors such as accommodation, transportation and health services, amongst others. RFPs may also contain information concerning the evaluation process. The RFP streamlines the bidding process so that the governing body can expect similar proposals from competing bidding cities.

Catherwood and Van Kirk (1992) point out that astute event bidders carefully analyze what is implied and what is required in an RFP. The governing body may not ask for certain rights or privileges, but the RFP may offer the opportunity to present them. This may present a strategy for bidding cities to "outdo" their competition wherever possible.

Event Bidding Process

Cities seeking to host international sport tourism events usually have to undertake an arduous bidding process. The bidding process for an Olympic Games will be reviewed to illustrate this point. Nine years prior to a given Olympics, the International Olympic Committee (IOC) formally invites National Olympic Committees (NOCs) to present candidate cities within six months. Serious candidate cities however have been preparing their bid well in advance of this deadline. As an NOC can nominate only one candidate city from its country, cities normally undergo a national bidding process. Major cities in South Africa, namely, Cape Town, Durban and Johannesburg, competed in a national bid to establish which city would go forward as South Africa's candidate city for South Africa. Once Cape Town was selected as the candidate city for South Africa, it had to submit a 10-minute presentation to the IOC Executive Board regarding its ability, support, and desire to host the Olympic Games. During this time, an information meeting is also held with the candidate cities so that they are aware of what is expected of them.

Bid Book Requirements

Each city receives a *Manual for Cities Bidding for the Olympic Games* from the IOC. As pointed out previously in this chapter, a manual was introduced in order to streamline the process so that all cities could be placed on equal footing when bidding for the Games. One essential requirement is the submission of the candidature file or *bid book*. It entails a synopsis of information required for 19 themes outlined by the *Manual*. The Cape Town 2004 bid book included the following themes:

1. National, regional, and candidate city characteristics
2. Legal aspects
3. Customs and immigration formalities
4. Environmental protection
5. Meteorological and environmental conditions
6. Security
7. Medical services
8. Program
9. General sports organization
10. Sports
11. Olympism and culture
12. Olympic village
13. Accommodation
13. Transport
14. Technology
15. Media
16. Finance
17. Marketing
18. Guarantees.

Although each event will have its own criteria, the themes gives one an understanding and framework for the bidding process.

IOC Evaluation Commission

Once the bid books have been submitted, the IOC assigns an evaluation commission to visit each city in order to discuss specifics regarding the bid based on the bid book submission. A technical report prepared by the commission is then sent to each IOC member. In the case of the 2004 Olympic Games' bidding process, 5 of the 11 cities were shortlisted as possible hosts. These 5 cities were then visited by the various IOC members before the final vote was taken. As part of the IOC policy reform in 1999, members are not permitted to make formal or informal visits to the cities submitting bids to host the Olympic Games.

Sport Tour: Five Still Alive as IOC Makes Cruelest Cut

Three European cities became front-runners to host the 2004 summer Olympic Games after the 11 original candidates were whittled down to 5 by the IOC's selection college. Athens, Rome, and Stockholm were joined by Cape Town and Buenos Aires. They had until September 1997 to polish their bids and deliver on key promises if they are to win the right to stage the greatest sporting show on earth. The announcement triggered a wave of joy among the successful city delegations. South African officials spoke of spontaneous street celebrations as the news of the decision was relayed to Cape Town. With economists' predictions that $1.7 billion in capital investment would be triggered by the Games and help boost the country's economic performance and create tens of thousands of jobs, Cape Town appeared to have more to gain than many. The decision sparked a new round of frenetic activity in a winner-takes-all battle that ended on 5 September 1997. (Source: Sport Business, 1997).

Final Presentation

Each city presents their bid at the IOC session at which the Olympic host city will be selected. The IOC members vote by secret ballot, and the city with a simple majority wins. This normally takes several rounds before a city gains a simple majority. In determining the host city for the 2004 Olympic Games, Rome lost out to Athens in the fifth and final round of voting, by a margin of 61 votes to 41 votes ("Ball Says," 1997). Once a new host city is selected, the city signs a "host city contract" with the IOC to ensure that the contractual obligations are carried out by the host city. On September 5, 1997, Athens was named host city for the 2004 Olympic Games.

The bidding process of the Olympic Games indicates the thoroughness required by candidate cities irrespective of the sport event. By addressing all the themes, the candidate city will be in a good position to ascertain whether all the issues have been examined. Critical to this process is the support generated by the community for the event.

Event Lobbying

Another important aspect of the bidding process is event lobbying. Bidding cities often put a lot of effort into discovering the identity of the real decision-makers. Catherwood and Van Kirk (1992) note that for many events, the members of a federation may defer the decision-making to a small, select group. In the case of the Olympic Games, behind-the-scenes lobbying, corruption, and bribery may occur as 104 International Olympic Committee (IOC) members vote to select the candidate city, as evidenced by the recent scandal surrounding the Salt Lake City Olympic bid.

Bidding Recommendations

Catherwood and Van Kirk (1992) recommend that the following four factors be considered in submitting a bid:

- Add quality control guarantees to the bid. The event must be thoroughly organized, and participants and officials are to receive quality treatment

- Propagate the event's main theme. IFs (International Federations) want to expand the influence of their sport

- Guaranteeing future fans equals better bidding potential. Spreading the sport creates a demand and a market

- Take advantage of a sole bidder position. Less popular sports have the advantage of not having as much competition, if any, compared to more popular sports

Planning Considerations

The planning process for sport tourism events can be a lengthy one. With increased competition for sport tourism events, the bidding and planning period is increasing. The planning process often begins with the idea to create a new event or to bid for an event that can be "won" for the community (Getz, 1997). Getz adds that tourism organizations are constantly on the lookout for events to win, especially when events have a parent or sponsoring organization, established track records, and local supporters. The preparation of a bid and a feasibility study can be incorporated in the planning process, or they can be viewed as quite separate tasks as we have done in this chapter. Although organizations engage in planning as a continuous process, one-time event organizations work towards a specific target completion. For annual or more permanent events to prosper, their planning should become more strategic by overcoming the tendency to plan each event as a new one.

A planning framework is required for regulated and accountable decision-making through policies, procedures, organizational structure, and evaluation (Getz, 1997). *Policies* are generally formal rules governing the activities of all members of the organization. They implement the mission and goals of the organization by showing what actions are desirable, permissible or forbidden. Within each policy field, procedures will be formulated to regulate routine action (Getz, 1997). Ultimately all decisions must be evaluated, and the decision-maker held accountable. Careful attention to organizational structure will help ensure that decisions are carefully made and fully implemented. Three aspects of planning, namely, the market plan, the business plan, and the strategic plan, will be dealt with in this chapter. The operations plan will be considered in chapter 9 as it is directly linked to the implementation strategies for the event.

Marketing may be defined simply as the set of organizational activities aimed at satisfying the customer. Marketing research includes the methods used by managers to know customer perceptions and expectations of service quality. A marketing philosophy refers to the social and economic justification for an organization's existence as the satisfaction of customer wants. The extent to which marketers make an effort to understand customer needs and expectations through formal and informal information-gathering activities is termed the *market research orientation* or philosophy. Knowing what customers expect is the first and probably the most important step in delivering quality service. Zeithaml, Parasuraman, and Berry (1990) underscore the importance of understanding customer expectations:

Being a little bit wrong about what customers want can mean losing a customer's business when another company hits the target exactly. Being a little bit wrong can mean expending money, time, and other resources on things that don't count to customers. Being a little bit wrong can even mean not surviving in a fiercely competitive market (p. 31)

Sometimes a gap exists between what sport tourists expect and what sport service providers perceive they expect. Because marketing research is a key vehicle for understanding customer expectations and perceptions of services, an organization that does not collect this information is more likely to experience this discrepancy.

Marketing research must focus on service quality issues, such as which features are most important to customers, which levels of these features customers expect, and what customers think the organization can and should do when problems occur in service delivery in order to close the gap.

Before a discussion of sport tourism marketing, it is important to know what customers expect in a service. Zeithaml et al. (1990) identified 10 components of service quality, each with implications to sport tourism marketing:

1. Tangibles: Appearance of physical facilities, equipment, personnel, and communication materials.

2. Reliability: Ability to perform the promised service dependably and accurately.

3. Responsiveness: Willingness to help customers and provide prompt service.

4. Competence: Possession of required skills and knowledge to perform the service.

5. Courtesy: Politeness, respect, consideration, and friendliness of contact person.

6. Credibility: Trustworthiness, believability, honesty of the service provider.

7. Security: Freedom from danger, risk, and doubt.

8. Access: Approachability and ease of contact.

9. Communication: Keeping customers informed in language they can understand and listening to them.

10. Understanding: Making an effort to know the customers and their needs.

From these 10 service quality elements, Zeithaml et al. identified five distinct dimensions, listed in order of importance to the customer:

1. Reliability: Ability to perform the promised service dependable and accurately.

2. Assurance: Knowledge and courtesy of employees and their ability to convey trust and confidence.

3. Responsiveness: Willingness to help customers and provide prompt service.

4. Empathy: Caring, individualized attention the agency provides its customers.

5. Tangibles: Appearance of physical facilities, equipment, personnel, and communication materials.

We may now have a clearer understanding of what service attributes are most important to sport tourists. Yet we also recognize that many "publics" (board members, organization executives, investors, political leaders, media, etc.) often have other service needs and requirements. For example, local politicians may be interested in the extent to which the sport tourism operation can create jobs for their constituencies whereas sport investors may be most interested in a financial return on investment. This is the first of several "reality checks" in this chapter. Answer the following questions as a market planner for a sport tourism organization:

• Who are our sport tourists?

• Why are others not consuming our services?

• How satisfied are customers with our services? How do you know?

- Which service attributes are most important to consumers and what do they think of our agency's performance on these variables?

- When do consumers decide to purchase our services or those of our competitors?

- What information is of most influence in consumers' decision-making process?

- Who are our direct competitors? What are our competitive advantages and shortcomings?

- What is the economic impact of our operations on the local economy? How much tax revenue is generated by our operations?

- What is the demand for and revenue potential of additional or expanded services?

There are several reasons why the sport tourism marketer may ask these questions. Below is a list of the possible reasons.

1. Measure consumer satisfaction.

2. Better serve consumers.

3. Justify marketing resource allocation decisions.

4. Identify and describe present/prospective markets and tailor marketing mix accordingly.

5. Determine promotional effectiveness.

6. Aid in securing/retaining sponsorship.

Primary market data collection can be an expensive and time-consuming project. As a result, many marketers opt to use secondary data resources to make promotional planning decisions. Sources of market research data include the Simmons Market Research Reports, National Sporting Goods Association, *Sport Market Place Annual*, and U.S. Bureau of the Census.

Market Segments

Consumer markets are most often segmented by geographic, demographic, and behavioral characteristics. Geographic descriptions are necessary but alone not sufficient for defining target markets. Boundaries for a neighborhood, city, and/or county are commonly used as geographic segment descriptors. Zip codes are often used rather than physical boundaries in determining geographic market segments. Travel times and geographical distance can also serve as useful variables for identifying potential user groups.

Demographic variables are measurable characteristics of a group or segment, such as age, gender, race, family size, education, occupation, and income levels. Customers belonging to the same demographic group may have common needs and interests and will demand certain services.

People who share geographic and demographic characteristics do not necessarily consume leisure services in the same manner. Therefore, behavioral variables, such as usage rate, stage of program consumption, skill level, and lifestyle, are important in determining target markets. Clients may be segmented by the extent to that a particular service is used. User categories may include some combination of the following: nonusers, former users, potential users, first-time users, light or irregular users, medium users, and heavy users.

Lifestyle or psychographic characteristics as a measure for target market segmentation measures people's activities in terms of how they spend their time and their view of themselves and the world around them. Psychographic segmentation groups people according to their lifestyle or personality traits.

Consumers may be segmented by the extent to which a particular sport is consumed. User categories may include some combination of the following: nonusers, former users, potential users, first-time users, light or irregular users, medium users, and heavy users. Mullin, Hardy, and Sutton (2000) developed the following continuum of sport user groups:

Uninterested—Nonaware—Media—Defector—Light User— Medium—Heavy User

Perhaps this example will illustrate why market segmentation is important. The spectator market for a winter sports festival may be segmented to include parents with small children and Generation Xers (among other segments). These segments may have some similar needs. However, they probably have more differences in terms of service expectations, requirements, and service quality perceptions. Parents and children may require clean changing tables in portable toilets, hard surfaces for strollers to easily maneuver throughout the grounds, puppet shows and clowns for entertainment, and admission price discounts for their young children. GenXers may only require progressive music at night. The point is, if we know what consumers want, services can be tailored accordingly. When services are provided at the highest quality, consumers may be satisfied and, in turn, tell others about how wonderful the services were.

For effective market segmentation, segments should be large enough to justify developing a specific marketing mix to service it, of a measurable size and accessible to distribution and communication efforts.

Two popular secondary data sources that provide lifestyle characteristics are VALS and PRIZM. Developed by Arthur Mitchell, SRI International, Values Attitudes and Lifestyles (VALS) sorts Americans into nine distinct categories based on their attitudes, personalities, and beliefs. Fees for market data range from a minimum $14,500 consultation to $110,000 for a one-year subscription to VALS Leading Edge social trends reports. Examples of VALS market segments are provided in the following section.

The Need Driven

Values Attitudes and Lifestyles (VALS)

Survivors. At the rock bottom of the economic ladder, these 6.8 million or 4% of the population may be the homeless, elderly and infirm or longtime welfare recipients; people who have fallen on hard times and have become trapped in a culture of poverty marked by despair and unhappiness.

Sustainers. Younger and slightly better off than the aforementioned, these 12 million (7% of the population) are the economically disadvantaged, but they have some hope for the future.

The Outer Directed

Belongers. The solid middle class (65 million Americans, 38% of the population) that defines American society is conservative and conformist. These people want to belong to families, groups, or clubs. They favor tradition and nostalgia. They tend to buy brand names and stable mass market items out of habit.

Emulators. The "wanna-be" yuppies—These competitive, very status conscious, upwardly mobile types (17.1 million, 10%) are conspicuous buyers. They rely heavily on what's in vogue.

Achievers. Formerly known as yuppies, this group (36 million, 20%) is the marketing gold mine. Achievers control nearly 50% of all consumer buying power in the United States. They are affluent types who have already arrived professionally and otherwise. They are ambitious, efficient, and comfort loving; they value success, fame, materialism, and the work ethic. They have the highest annual household income and tend to hold technical or professional jobs.

The Inner Directed

I-Am-Me's. These 5.1 million Americans (3% of the population) are the young, highly individualistic vanguard. They are experimental, impulsive, and self-expressive.

Experientials: These 8.6 million (5%) constitute the slightly older crowd, but no less committed to gaining life experiences than the "I-Am-Me"s. They are individualistic, avant-garde, and artistic. Jogging, using VCRs, and eating health foods and granola all started among this group.

Societally conscious. This group (20.5 million, 11%) has a sense of social responsibility. They are activists, highly educated, involved in conservation, environmental, and consumer movements. They value authenticity and inner growth.

The Integrated. They (3.4 million, 2%) are the most elite of the market segments, composed of exceptional business and social leaders and innovators.

PRIZM

PRIZM is another market segmentation system based on the principle that people with similar backgrounds, means, and consumer behavior cluster in neighborhoods suited to their lifestyles. PRIZM may be accessed through the home page for parent company, Claritas Express: www.delluke.claritas.com:80/Express/clxhome.wjsp. Through a complex statistical analysis of its demographic characteristics and actual consumer behavior, every U.S. neighborhood, over 500,00 in all, is assigned to one of the 40 PRIZM clusters. Below are two brief examples of PRIZM clusters.

Blue Blood Estates

	What They Like	And Don't Like
Automobiles	Jaguar	Monte Carlo
Investments	Treasury Notes	Christmas Club
Leisure/Sports	Skiing	Pro Wrestling
Package Goods	Frozen Pastry	TV Dinners
Vacation/Travel	Foreign Travel	Camper/Trailer

New Melting Pot

	What They Like	And Don't Like
Automobiles	Mitsubishi	Ford Escort
Investments	Cert. of Deposit	Credit Unions
Leisure/Sports	Horse Racing	Hunting
Package Goods	Yogurt	Pizza Mixes
Vacation/Travel	Railway	Cruise Ships

Target Markets

Crompton and Lamb (1986) define a target market as a relatively homogeneous group of people with relatively similar service preferences with which the agency seeks to do business. They describe the importance of this stage in the market planning process:

The identification and selection of target market groups influences and often directly determines all of the ensuing decisions that must be made regarding types of services, their distribution, pricing, and communication. Once target markets have been identified, everything the agency does must be tailored to the wants of the people in these groups. (p. 112)

Markets for sport tourism services are composed of people with wants and needs for particular programs and services who possess the ability and desire to purchase/use these programs and services. Determining the target markets to which a service should be offered is a two-stage process. The first stage is concerned with identifying all of the heterogeneous groups in a market, each of which may be a potential target market. The second stage is to select which of these potential client groups the agency intends to serve with a particular service. The marketing executive must decide whose needs to serve before deciding what needs to serve.

Sport Tourist Destination Area (STDA) Characteristics

In order to gain a better understanding of planning for a sport tourism event, it is necessary to consider it within a broader context of planning for a sport tourism destination area. What produces a positive sport tourism image for a community? Attractions are the first order for any sport tourist destination area. Accessibility to the destination by visitors is essential. Effective communications are also important as sport tourists obviously do not go to places they have not heard about. Accommodations, such as lodging, shops, and eating and drinking places, are tourism support services. Hospitality is a component of a community's tourism image that is often underemphasized. Sport tourists go where they are invited and stay where they feel welcome. They will also tell others about how well or poorly they were treated by hosts. Word-of-mouth referrals are among the most effective promotional methods for sport tourism destination areas.

Types of Sport Tourism Resources

1. Natural tourism resources: Terrain, climate, geology, water, flora, fauna.
2. Manmade tourism resources: Historical/cultural, hospitality facilities, sport/recreation facilities, events, and experiences.
3. Human tourism resources: Hosting capabilities, provision of human services, aspects of ambient culture.
4. Community location: With regard to physical resources and market access, a distinct, exploitable factor in tourism potential.

Not every community is an STDA, but with planning, adequate resource allocations, and proper implementation, a community can become an attractive sport tourism locale. The essential elements of a sport tourist destination area:

1. A recognized, definable appeal to travelers.

2. A tourism identity of sufficient scale to deserve treatment as a factor in the local economy.

3. Coherence in its geography and among its tourist-related features.

4. Political integrity so that viable decisions can be made.

5. Communication/information distribution channels.

6. Access to the destination (modes of transportation and accessible transportation corridors).

7. Residents willing to accept/embrace tourism.

8. Defined attractions.

9. Accommodation and service employees.

Sport tourism resources are considered any factor, natural or man-made, tangible or intangible, that is available to attract and contribute positively to tourists' experience in a community.

I. Getting Started

The first step in maximizing a community's sport tourism potential is to assemble the "players" in the sport tourism industry. These leaders may include representatives from

Attractions:	Parks and recreation department executive, outdoor resource managers, owners of selected commercial attractions
Accommodations:	Hotel/motel association president
Retail shopping:	Downtown association president, chamber of commerce president
Transportation:	County transportation officer
Government:	Economic development executive, convention and visitors bureau director
Promotion:	Travel agency presidents

II. Intelligence Gathering

To accurately respond to the questions posed in a strategic plan's SWOT analysis, market research must be conducted. SWOT refers to an assessment of a sport organization's Strengths, Weaknesses, Opportunities, and Threats. Data on sport tourism markets may be obtained from sport-governing bodies, national sport organizations, census data, or other secondary sources. Other information sources include the *Journal of Sport Tourism, Journal of Travel Research, Annals of Tourism Research*, and the Travel and Tourism Research Association.

III. Action Planning

Action strategies describe the specific activities to be taken to achieve sport tourism planning initiatives and identification of the people who will carry them out. Guidelines should be developed providing a written description of each target market and sport tourism service, the needs of each target market to be met by each service, the selected marketing mix, and service standards.

Sport Tourism Development Action Strategies

- *Target Markets: Define sport tourism target markets geographically, demographically, and in attitudinal and behavioral terms.*
- *Attractions: Describe each sport tourism attraction (core, peripheral, supplemental) to be offered and "packaged" during the planning period, and justify its existence.*
- *Needs: State the needs of each targeted sport tourism market to be fulfilled by each service.*
- *Objectives: Specify operational objectives for each sport tourism initiative.*
- *Price: State overall pricing policy (i.e., free, subsidized, going rate, etc.) and assess cost-benefit ratios.*
- *Distribution: Specify service location and scheduling in relation to targeted markets.*
- *Promotion: Describe and justify the promotional strategies for each sport tourism market.*
- *Service: Determine the service standards that have been established and how they are monitored.*

Source: J. L. Crompton & C. W. Lamb, Marketing government and social services. New York: John Wiley & Sons, 1986, p. 66.

Business Planning Considerations

Getz (1997) contends that the most common reason for preparing a business plan is to obtain financing. Moreover, it is perhaps the most direct route to finding investors to generate the start-up capital required for the event (Graham et al., 1997). There are a number of other reasons for preparing an updating a business plan, as outlined by Getz (1997), and they include the following:

- To obtain financing from sponsors, lenders, and grant-givers.

- To demonstrate management competency to all stakeholders, including staff and volunteers.

- To facilitate partnerships and alliances.

- To make clear the organization's aims, objectives, and priorities.

- To get started on a project and to attract key people.

- To establish sound financial planning and control mechanisms.

A comprehensive business plan includes key points concerning background on the organization of the event, plans for developing and improving the event, marketing and communications strategies, and financial management plans. A case for financial assistance can be made if required. Business plans are useful in strategic planning and budgeting. The exercise of developing and updating the business plan will tend to force higher levels of management competency on the organization and lead to better cost-revenue management.

Once the plan has been prepared, prospective sponsors to invest in the event have to be approached. There are number of sources such as the *Sports Marketplace* and the *Sports Sponsors Fact Book* that can assist in preparing you with your search for sponsors. Other marketing references such as *IEG Sponsorship Report* and *Advertising Age* can identify corporations that understand the rewards of investing in sport events.

Strategic Planning Considerations

The literature abounds with definitions of strategic planning. The following definition sums up the process:

Strategic planning is the process of determining an organization's long-term goals and objectives in compliance with its mission and formulating the proper plan of action (strategy), policies and programs that insure that sound decisions will be made about internal resources and environmental factors that affect all effort to achieve the desired end results over the long run. (Bridges & Roquemore, 1992, p. 88)

The significance of current processes that affect the changing organization in the future and the effectiveness and efficiency of plans and programs to meet organizational goals and objectives is intrinsic to the strategic planning process. The mission statement and the organizational aims and objectives are generally recognized as the first two components of this process.

Identifying the Sport Tourism Event's Mission Statement

A mission statement is a broad, visionary focus that explains what the organization wants to accomplish. The reasons that an organization wishes to achieve its goals are related to its mission statement; therefore, the mission statement focuses the direction of all effort.

Identifying Sport Tourism Event Aims and Objectives

It is absolutely essential to identify the aims of the event at the earliest stage. One is required to have a clear understanding of the event and predict the rewards. Once the aims have been established, it will be necessary to set more manageable objectives. Organizational objectives are more detailed statements derived from the mission statement. They should be able to be converted into specific plans at an operational level (Davis, 1994). In so doing, the objectives can be more easily quantified, and their progress can be measured (Bridges & Roquemore, 1992). Bridges and Roquemore further conclude that the purpose of strategic planning is to formulate long-term objectives.

It is vital that all stakeholders understand and agree on the objectives in order to ensure a greater commitment to achieving the targets. The precise definition of objectives further assists in establishing an organizational structure. It allows each individual or committee to be given a number of targets that they are responsible for attaining (Watt, 1992). It also reflects the need for cooperation as many objectives will more than likely be interdependent. Objectives set should be realistic, simple, clear, unambiguous, and achievable (Watt). The following key objectives were cited by the 8th World Swimming Championships Organizing Committee, which was held in Perth in January 1998:

1. To successfully develop and manage a World Championships event of the highest international standard.

2. To provide the best conditions for competitors and officials and to present the highest level of international competition to a worldwide audience.

3. To promote the benefits of swimming, water polo, diving, synchronized swimming and open water swimming to international, national and state communities.

4. To manage the event with the approved budget while maximizing the commercial opportunities available to all stakeholders.

5. To effectively raise and promote the sport, cultural and tourism profiles of Perth, Western Australia and Australia.

6. To demonstrate Western Australia and Australia's ability to stage major international sporting events through the coordinated involvement of government, the private sector, sports organizations, the media, commercial organizations and volunteer support groups. (Melchert, 1997, p. 4)

SWOT Analysis

Once the mission statement, aims, and objectives have been identified and defined, the next step for more permanent events is to review existing strategy. A useful test to evaluate the need to change strategy is to determine whether performance meets objectives (Bridges & Roquemore, 1992). Any significant difference would suggest a review of existing strategy. For new events, the most appropriate strategies will have to be identified. A SWOT analysis is an essential consideration in the planning phase as it assists in identifying the internal and external variables that prevent the proposed event from achieving maximum success (Goldblatt, 1997). This analysis consists of identifying the strengths (S) and weaknesses (W) of the proposed event plan and the opportunities (O) and threats (T) to the event. Strengths and weaknesses can be identified prior to the event. Existing and potential market must be identified, and competitors and complementary events and sport tourism event products, evaluated, leading to identification of opportunities and threats (Getz, 1997). Opportunities and threats generally present themselves during or after the event (Goldblatt). Weakness should be eliminated or minimized, and attempts should be made in the event planning phase to increase the strengths.

Activities that present themselves without significant investment from the event organization may be considered opportunities. For example, in an attempt to identify the target market for a sport tourism event, existing research on consumer market segments as discussed previously during market planning can be considered an opportunity. Threats are those conditions that prevent one from maximizing the potential of the proposed event (Goldblatt, 1997). Inclement weather and political infighting may be considered threats to the success of the event. Terrorism and high crime rates are factors that further need to be considered as they may prevent individuals from attending. The drug-testing saga that occurred at the 1998 Tour de France may be considered a threat to the success of future races. It is, therefore, essential to consider threats very carefully, and ways should be found to contain, reduce, or eliminate potential threats.

The SWOT analysis is a useful tool that assists the organizers in scanning the internal and external environment. Moreover, weaknesses and threats can be analyzed so that solutions can be provided to improve the event planning process (Goldblatt, 1997). Competitive advantages can be further isolated. Clearly, research undertaken in the initial stages is critical to producing an effective event because it provides an opportunity to determine whether one has the necessary internal and external resources. Moreover, the SWOT analysis is central to other types of planning as

Sport Tour: Vodacom Beach Africa

The Vodacom Beach Africa Festival Durban (as opposed to the Ocean Action Festival) arose out of the annual Gunston 500 International Surfing Championships (now known as the Mr Price Pro). In the 1990s, Durban Tourism realized that this major surfing event has a extraordinary impact on Durban, as thousands of local and international sport tourists flocked to Durban each year to share in this event. Durban Tourism felt that by adding additional events and activities, they could attract even more people to the championship and create a substantial increase in tourism expenditure over that period. In 1993, this idea developed into one of the world's largest sand and surf festivals, held annually between the 10th and 20th of July in Durban. The activities, besides the world-renowned Gunston 500, include both competitive and recreational activities such as

- Korfbal development
- Agfa Beach Soccer Challenge
- Scott Little Miss SPCA.
- RCI Night Surfing Skins Event (world-class field of national and international competitors).
- Spiced Gold (live bands in the entertainment marquee)
- Skateboard ramp (open to public)
- Clover Roadshows
- Ocean Action/SPCA Grand Opening Parade
- Alpha Strongman (public demonstrations with strongmen Pieter de Bruyn and Gerrit Badenhorst)
- McDonald's National Inflatable Boat Contest
- Smirnoff International Areobatic Team
- Iron Man & Diamond Lady Events & Surfboat Challenge
- Combat Group Longboard Pro
- Wakeboarding Demonstrations
- July in the Entertainment Marquee—Fashion shows with Roberta Alessandri Models
- Ola Queen of the Beach Volleyball
- Take 5 Roadshows
- Bourbon Street Ladies Night
- Body-painting—in the entertainment marquee
- Coca-Cola Body Board Classic
- Neal Stephenson Fund Mass Paddle
- Gunston 500
- Live Music presented by SA Brewers—in the entertainment marquee
- Clairwood Party by the Sea
- Nandos/Health & Racquet Fitness Challenge
- Surf Obsession/Glodina Development Bodyboarding Contest
- Miss Mini Clover
- Flying Crunchie—amazing stunt flying
- Mainstay King of the Surf Jetski Challenge
- Miss Pick 'n Pay Hypermarket/Mystery Teen Ocean Action
- Alpha Strongman South African Championships
- Red Bull Skateboarding Challenge
- Beach Volleyball National Champions Tournament (men's & women's event)
- Olive Computers Canoe Polo
- Bernini Beach Touch Rugby
- Miss Southern Comfort Ocean Action
- Bluff Meat Supply Kick-Boxing Extravaganza.

What started out as a surfing event has attracted family holidaymakers in addition to the surfing crowd. The 2000 festival attracted a volume of over 900,000 visitors and generated in excess of R500 million (about US$62 million) for the City of Durban over the 10-day period.

Source: Wholisitc Consulting and Development in collaboration with the Department of Geography and Environmental Studies, University of Durban Westville.

well. For example, when discussing the sport tourism destination areas (STDA) earlier in this chapter, it is possible to identify many of the necessary characteristics and role players essential to maximizing a community's sport tourism potential on the basis of a SWOT analysis.

Situational Analysis

A situational analysis is very similar to the SWOT analysis. Getz (1997) contends that a "situational analysis" is equivalent to taking stock of the organization and its environment. He further suggests that such an analysis has several components:

1. Environmental scanning—seeks to identify conditions and underlying forces shaping events and event tourism.

2. Future scanning—extends trends into the future to assess the probability and potential impacts of future conditions.

3. Resource appraisals—examines the availability of human, financial, political and material support to meet the event's goals.

Scanning must, therefore, include economic, social, cultural, ecological, political, and technological forces and trends (Getz, 1997). Public input, through formal surveys, focus groups, or public forums, will assist this process. The public should be consulted on their attitudes toward the organization and towards events and tourism in general (Getz, 1997). Government tourism and social trends data as well as other pertinent research material should be reviewed (Getz, 1997). Getz (1997) further states that it could be advantageous to commission a study of trends and forces shaping events and tourism in your area.

Strategy Formulation, Implementation, and Evaluation

A number of issues will arise from the background research and analysis. Strategy formulation will assist in dealing with these issues. The strategy that

---

Sport Tour: Tour de France Doping Scandal

To say that the sport of cycling is in a crisis is a weak understatement at best. Police continued to search the vehicles and hotel rooms and luggage of professional teams and riders at the Tour de France, and French, Belgian, Dutch and Swiss courts stepped up their investigations into drug-related activities in cycling. The ramifications of the "Tour de France doping scandal" are potentially fatal to cycling, Sponsors—even those who have public professed their support for cycling—may eventually be scared away. Fans, including those who stand for hours on the sides of the narrow Belgian lanes, cobbled French roads, or the fog-enshrouded mountain passes of the Alps and the Pyrenees, just to catch a glimpse of their favorite riders, could eventually find other interests. And young riders, already dwindling in numbers in the United States, could easily be discouraged from participating in a sport tainted by drugs. The sport itself is at risk. Despite Lance Armstrong's Tour victories in 1999 and 2000, questions continue about whether he and/or other members of the U.S. Postal Service Team used banned performance enhancing substances.

is finally accepted should be one that meets the degree of risk that the organization deems acceptable (Bridges & Roquemore, 1992). Every strategy should further be accompanied by a time horizon. Once an alternative strategy is selected, plans are developed to provide direction to the organization (Bridges & Roquemore). Plans consist of programs, policies, and procedures. Bruntland (1988) asserts that action plans should be presented in written form and should include expected results and realistic project realization dates.

The final step in the strategic planning process is the implementation and control of the strategy. Once the component plans and programs are initiated, the strategy is activated. Strategies will be required for each of the management function. Feasibility studies and cost-benefit evaluations should be used to determine the viability of a strategy, and failure to involve all stakeholders will minimize efficient implementation of strategies (Getz, 1997).

Getz (1997) recommends that the following principles be followed to ensure that plans will be implemented:

- Develop a shared vision that all stakeholders can accept.

- Maximize stakeholder involvement in the entire process.

- Develop strategies instead of blueprints.

- Focus on results and how to attain and evaluate them.

- Develop action plans with timelines and assigned responsibilities.

In addition to the crucial research efforts mentioned above, a comprehensive evaluation system must be established. Evaluation is a critical part of control. Bridges and Roquemore (1992) describe control as the function of measuring actual performance against the expected results or the desired results. The strategy should be evaluated to ascertain whether the strategy is being implemented as designed (Bridges & Roquemore). Moreover, strategic choices often require modification to the organization, such as its committee structure or its organizational roles, to ensure implementation (Getz, 1997).

Schaffir (1988) concludes that to get value from strategic planning, the focus should be on strategic thinking and doing as opposed to merely generating planning-related paper-work as evidenced in the conventional approach. Moreover, people are considered the link between a strategy and its success. Strategy implementation is thus a part of everyone's job. A contemporary approach calls for a planning process that is fluid, flexible, and open to change. It is important to note that as the dynamics of the sport market place are shifting so rapidly, an organization will more than likely benefit from strategic planning only if it remains flexible to the changing environment. Furthermore, it is evident from the above discussions that market, business, and strategic planning for a sport tourism events are inextricably linked. In addition, one cannot discuss these aspects without consideration for planning of the sport tourism destination area (STDA) as a whole.

Organizational Structure

The organizational structure assists in determining the activities to be accomplished towards achieving the objectives of the event and allocating the achievement of objectives through these activities to the appropriate groups or individuals (Watt, 1992). Likewise Getz (1997) asserts that without formulation of goals and strategies, an inappropriate organizational structure might be created. In addition, starting with a business plan, including a sound budget and cash-flow projections, will place the organization on firm footing (Getz, 1997). Advocating a structure, defining who does what, is a key consideration for all events. Determining the appropriate type of structure and having it formally organized is a matter of planning, consultation with experts, and perhaps trial and error (Getz, 1997). There is no one best way to structure an event organization, as the size of the structure will depend on the level, complexity, and nature of the event.

A simple organizational structure is depicted in the figure below as an example for smaller scale sport tourism events.

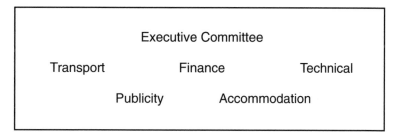

Figure 4.1. A Simple Organizational Structure

Major events require a more complex organization chart. The organizational chart of the 8th World Swimming Championships is depicted on the next page as representative of this type of organizational structure.

In order to further elucidate the complexity of a major sporting event, the organizational structure can be further defined by the administration it entails as indicated in the administration organizational chart of the 8th World Championships Organizing Committee (Melchert, 1997). Melchert further notes that position on the chart does not necessarily indicate level within the organization.

Event Staff	SECRETARIAT	Consultants
(Volunteers)	Contractors	

8th World Swimming Championships Sub Committees

Diving	Special Events
Open Water Swimming	Technology
Swimming	Transport
Synchronized Swimming	Venue Management
Water Polo	Volunteer Services
Accommodation	Welcome, Entertainment & Hospitality
Accreditation	
Ceremonial	Chairpersons
Liaison	FINA—Federation Internationale Natation, International Swimming Federation
Marketing	
Media	
Medical	ASI—Australian Swimming Institute

Figure 4.2. FINA 8th World Swimming Chamionships Organization

Wilkinson (1988) suggests that a successful organizational structure can be achieved in the following ways:

1. Delimit the levels of authority and responsibility, and ensure that these levels are distinctly outlined.

2. Delimit the number of managers, coordinators, and committee sizes.

3. Formulate written job descriptions for each individual.

4. Keep your organizational structure simple.

The structure of the event is the principal step in the management of the activities that will lead to a successful event. However, as pointed out by Wilkinson, the evolution of an organizational chart by itself will not create a successful event. It will, nevertheless, make the prerequisites for success more clearly identified. Once the overall structure is established, it is essential to set down detailed parameters for each individual or group. Each person must be quite clear about his or her particular responsibilities in order to ensure smooth coordination and communication within the event organizational structure.

Minister of Sport and Recreation Organizing Committee

Chairman	Executive Secretary		
Executive Director	Executive Assistant		
Receptionist (2)	Sports and Operations Director		
Marketing Director	Operations Manager		
Accommodation & Accreditation	PA Secretary	Volunteers	Media
Event Support Co-ord	Supervisor	Staff co-ord	Manager
WP/Clerk (2)			
Accommodation	Accreditation	Volunteer	Media Liaison
Assistant (5) — Assistant (2)	Assistant (2)	Co-ord	
PA/Secretary — Marketing	Sports Co-ord	WP/Clerk (2)	Media
Hospitality Co-ord — (5 Disciplines)		Assistant (3)	
Catering — Marketing	Liaison Co-ord		
Co-ord — Assistant (3)			
Operations			
Assistant (3)			

Figure 4.3. Example of a Sport Tourism Organizational Structure

Project Management Team

To accentuate flexibility and communications, it is suggested that the project management team incorporate a "flat" structure as opposed to a bureaucratic hierarchy. The project management team usually consists of an executive director and a magnitude of functional area managers, depending on the character of the project. The project manager will require skills and experience in event project management. A fundamental qualification is the manager's ability to organize, motivate, and manage a team of experts and volunteers. Planning and team building are the focus of the first stage of project management. Thereafter, control becomes the main management task. The bid stage might well require its own project team. It is not unusual for major sport tourism events to have a different team once the bid has been won. Production of the event often requires a different set of skills from those needed in the early stages. The team, therefore, will usually have a built-in transition of people with the appropriate skills of planning, control, and production.

Timeline Considerations

Attention to the timeline is required as early as the feasibility study. Critical path analysis and program evaluation and review techniques (PERT) are two planning and scheduling tools that can assist in streamlining the planning process. Critical path analysis examines the interrelationships among all the stakeholders and activities required to deliver the event as intended (Getz, 1997). All tasks are arranged in chronological order, working back from the event dates, so that each essential activity is scheduled in the relevant order. When all the tasks are linked and critical dates (i.e., dates by which the tasks are to be completed) fixed, a line can be drawn to clarify how long at a minimum the process will take and how various pieces fit together. Separate exercises could be undertaken for the different program areas, venues, or specific activities related to the event and then brought together at key points in the network diagram (Getz, 1997).

PERT is similar to critical path analysis, but instead of working back from a fixed date its basis is the identification of minimum, most likely, and projected timelines (Getz, 1997). Getz (1997) adds that this approach is more suited to events that do not have to be produced on a specific schedule. PERT permits prediction of the final complete date or of milestones on the path to a fixed event date. For one-time events, predicting the full number of tasks and the likely schedule may be difficult. PERT can thus be employed to estimate project timelines and determine the feasibility of the event. In most instances, however, once a commitment is made, the project team must get it done, no matter what. This pressure leads to a number of issues as outlined by Getz (1997):

- The requirement for fast-tracking—Governments agree to suspend or modify various regulations to ensure completion.

- Increased expenditure—As the deadline looms, more money may have to be spent for overtime work and for outsourcing work.

- Sacrifices in quality—Plans may have to be altered with a resultant reduction in quality.

- Need for revision—Plan revisions might be required regularly, and without satisfactory assessments of impacts.

- Increased susceptibility to external forces, such as protests, or to internal forces such as labor disputes.

- Public relations problems, particularly if it appears that the project is behind schedule or is being reduced in quality or scope.

- Scheduling and controlling are, therefore, critical management responsibilities that necessitate careful consideration.

Many events have specific physical dimensions; therefore, careful considerations of their setting and location are required.

Setting and Location Considerations

Setting

Getz (1997) identified six generic event settings, namely, assemblies, processions, linear-nodal, open space, exhibition/sales, and activities. The suitability of a specific setting will be related to the aims and the program of the event.

The emphasis in assemblies settings is on the preparation of efficient, comfortable, and enjoyable viewing and listening, which are the prerequisites of most conventions, formal ceremonies, and spectator sports. Present facilities with their own management systems can be used (e.g., exposition halls, auditoriums. and arenas). Processions, including parades, are linear, mobile kinds of entertainment with distinct design and management stipulations. The audience might be standing, seated, or moving along with the procession. However, the most common linear setting is a street with a static audience along the route. Some processions pass through seating areas and stadia and take on the appearance of theater.

Many sport events involve races or other linear forms of activity. Long-distance multi-sport events, which combine procession with nodes of activity, for example, triathlons, duathlons, and biathlons, are also common. The audience generally gathers at the nodes, such as start, finish, and transition points. Events with open-space settings often use parks, plazas and closed streets. An essential characteristic of these settings is free movement, but they usually contain subareas for assembly, procession, and exhibition/sales.

Exhibition/sales settings are planned to lure entry and circulation, browsing and sales. Occasionally, the audience merely views the exhibits; in others, sales are made on the spot. For example, visitors to the National Football League Hall of Fame may view exhibits and purchase memorabilia in the retail shop, whereas baseball card collectors may browse, purchase, and trade cards with vendors at card shows. Food and beverage concessions are often presented in this manner. Sports and other activities frequently require purpose-built facilities, although many can be combined with other settings. The type of sport event and facility availability within the host region may limit venue selection. Most events require a range of support spaces and facilities, and the necessity for any of these will in part determine the suitability of the setting.

Location

A number of significant conditions, such as visibility, accessibility, centrality, and clustering, amongst others, should be considered (Getz, 1997). High visibility may be an essential factor in choosing event location for attracting customers, particularly for open-air events and parades. Moreover, certain types of events want high visibility for the media, rather than for on-site audiences. For example, determination of the photogenic backdrop and optimal broadcasting viewpoints will be factors in choosing a parade route. Many races require special types of beginning, ending, and transition points. Getz (1997) contends that the more spontaneous the decision to attend, the more likely it is that visibility will influence customers. Passersby, as well as those in attendance, should be able to see some of the event's ambiance and attractions.

Accessibility, in terms of how customers reach the event, will also help ascertain suitable locations. Consideration should be given to various means of transport, such as car, bus or train, as well as the volume and timing of each type. Furthermore, the location should be able to handle surplus demand, such as adequate provision of additional parking areas. Shuttle services from parking areas or public transport stations are recommended if accessibility is anticipated to be a problem (Getz, 1997). Easy connections to airports, freeways, and public transport terminals are essential when targeting tourists.

Getz (1997) asserts that to maximize factors such as accessibility and visibility, a central location within a community is often preferred. He recommends geographical analysis to be performed to determine how central and accessible various locations are, relative to target markets. Other considerations may be political or symbolic. For example, politicians may favor central locations close to or using civic facilities, whereas the business community might favor main streets or shopping centers.

Clustering is the association of events with other attractions and services (Getz, 1997). Centrality often results in clustering. Events on a city waterfront or within the tourist business district will probably maximize clustering and, therefore, offer the customer more to see and do in the area. This is especially true for tourists who may not know about the event in advance and may gravitate to areas where attractions, services, and events are concentrated (Getz, 1997).

The appropriateness of the location has to be determined as well. For example, parades and community festivals often require streets to be closed off. Consideration of whether a safety hazard will be created or businesses on the street will be likely to suffer is required. Public parks may appear to be easy choices; however, certain activities may not be appropriate for all parks. Therefore, an EIA, as outlined previously, is essential in determining location.

Cost may be an additional factor in choosing a location. Related costs, such as security or utilities, can be affected by the location of the event.

Furthermore, cost to consumers in terms of driving time, transport, and parking charges should be considered.

Free Versus Paid Admission	Schmader and Jackson (1997) contend that the events industry in general is divided on the issue of whether to charge admission to programs or to offer them free to the public. Some argue that the public perceives free events as inferior and, therefore, will not attend. Purchased tickets are often used as a way to control spectator attendance. However, distribution of only a certain allocation of free tickets can serve the same purpose (Schmader & Jackson). It appears that free attendance does not hurt attendance, and events generally do well if they are well sponsored, well produced, and well marketed. If one decides to sell tickets, one must ensure that the price is equitable to what is being offered. Noting what the market will accept as reasonable for comparable events may be useful.

Factors Related to Poor Events	Often, after years and years of doing the same thing without adding any fresh elements, a successful event can turn out to be mediocre. It is, therefore, important to consider a number of factors that can prevent one from producing a high-quality event. The conscientious sport tourism event organizer will work hard to avoid these pitfalls.

1. Insufficient Creativity and Innovation

Schmader and Jackson (1997) report that many event organizations duplicate theme events because there is a lack of creative application. For an event to stand out on a national, or even a regional, level, it must be different from and better than others must. An effort must be made to be innovative so that the event is distinctive. Annual events may suffer as a result of complacency.

2. Indifferent Marketing

The appearance of the marketing material is an indication of the quality of the overall marketing program. A new event, especially, must be expertly marketed because it does not have the word-of-mouth publicity to build interest in it. Even established events must constantly improve their marketing techniques.

3. Incompetent Personnel

It is important to ensure that the paid as well as volunteer staff are adequately prepared and qualified for their allocated positions. Too few events have effective training and recruiting programs for volunteers.

4. Too Much, Too Often

Many events compromise their quality by attempting to offer too much. Concentrate on just a few events and make sure that they are of a high standard.

5. Insufficient Funding

As pointed out in earlier in the discussion of the feasibility study, securing funding is of vital importance to the success of the event. It is sometimes better to abort an event, rather than try to persist when it is apparent that inadequate funding will result in a failure. However, it is important to note that not all events need a phenomenal amount of funding to be successful, especially at a local level (Watt, 1992).

6. Poor Timing

The feasibility study should identify the best schedule for the proposed event. Enough time should be allowed between the feasibility study and the actual event. If human or financial resources are lacking, consider having the event every second year instead of annually. Timing in relation to the weather should also be considered. For example, if an event is constantly rained out, then obviously, a more suitable date should be sought. Timing is also essential when considering the actual program of activity. An attempt should be made at setting enough time aside for the activities for the day and not spreading too few over a couple of days.

7. Inferior Physical Environment

Planning is crucial to prevent problems such as insufficient parking, traffic congestion, inadequate stadia and malfunctioning scoreboards. These issues should be closely monitored throughout the event.

Future Considerations

It is evident that hosting sport tourism events as a strategy can be easy for communities to initiate. However, because the competition is intense, hosting the appropriate event requires a high degree of professionalism and investment. It is recommended, therefore, that communities focus on a particular strategy instead of bidding on or hosting whatever sport tourism event comes along. Therefore, the community will need to develop a portfolio of sport tourism events.

Getz (1998) suggests the following strategies to assist communities in the portfolio-building process:

1. Creating new events: In order to find competitive advantages, communities, together with sporting bodies and tourism agencies can act

to create new events with the potential to attract large numbers and/ media attention.

2. Pursuing participant events: This strategy concentrates mainly on attracting individual athletes to participate in activities such as fun runs and open tournaments. The advantage of this type of event is that sport-governing bodies are not necessarily involved. Moreover, these events often attract family and friends for additional leisure experiences in the destination.

3. Pursuing media events: Media events can be considered as those events that attract sponsors and media coverage but do not necessarily attract large crowds. These events have excellent potential to provide publicity without the requirement of hosting large numbers of visitors. However, Getz (1998) cautions that hosting the media can present its own set of challenges.

4. Cultivating a niche: In order for communities to find a competitive advantage, they can elect to focus on a particular type of event or sport such as sports requiring a specific kind of venue. In so doing, a community can develop an appropriate and attractive portfolio of sport tourism events in which the occasional mega-event is balanced by bidding on lesser occasional events and periodic local or regional-scale events (Getz, 1998). Clearly, communities that can never aspire to hosting a major sport tourism event can still capitalize on sport tourism by carving out a suitable niche in hosting small-scale amateur events.

Summary

Although the hosting of sport tourism events can be a very challenging project to embark upon, careful consideration needs to be given to a myriad of details in order for a successful event to be staged. Research and planning are two vital steps in designing a sport tourism event. Market planning, business planning, and strategic planning are critical considerations in designing sport tourism events This initial stage is indeed important as it prepares the host organization for transition to event implementation and, finally, event shutdown.

When one considers hosting an event, one will be required to convince the owner of the event that one has the capability of successfully conducting the event. In some cases, this requires a formal bidding process, which, for major international events, can be an arduous procedure.

It is vitally important that the uniqueness of the event be recognized and although there are basic considerations that can be applied to designing successful events, each event should not treated as the same.

Once-prosperous events become mediocre for many reasons. Cognizance should be taken of the factors contributing to the poor quality so that such events may be re-energized.

In lieu of the increased competition to host sport tourism events, it may be beneficial for communities to build up a portfolio of sport tourism events, as suggested by Getz (1998), in order to carve a niche in the sport tourism market.

---

1. Why do some people leave home to attend or participate in sport?

2. Describe how you would select the most appropriate event for your community and discuss some of the most important determinants used to reach this decision.

3. Review an event previously held in your community, and on the basis of a SWOT analysis, identify ways in which the design of the event can be improved.

4. Given that community support is often a neglected factor in designing sport tourism events, what strategies would you use to seek community support and what groups would you involve?

5. Using Getz's (1998) strategy for selecting a sport tourism event portfolio, identify and justify the strategy most appropriate for your community.

Recommended Readings

Ahmed Z. U., Krohn, F. B., and Heller, V.L. (1997). World University Games—1993 at Buffalo (New York): Boosting Its Tourism Industry or Missing an Opportunity—An International Marketing Perspective. *Journal of Professional Services Marketing, 14* (2), 79–97.

Bramwell, B. (1997). Strategic planning before and after a mega-event. *Tourism Management, 18* (3), 167–176.

Hall, C. M. (1992). *Hallmark Tourist Events, Impacts, Management and Planning.* London: Bellhaven.

Hall, C. M. (1996). Hallmark Events and Urban Reimaging Strategies. Coercion, Community and the Sydney 2000 Olympics. Practicing Responsible Tourism. In Harrison, L. C. and Husbands, W. (Eds.), *International Case Studies in Tourism, Planning, Policy, and Development* pp. 336–379). New York: Wiley.

Sport Tourism in the Barbados—The Development of Sports Facilities and Special Events. (1997, April). *Journal of Sport Tourism* [Online], 4(1). Available: www.free-press.com/journals/jst/ [1998, February 5].

Weed, M. E. and Bull, C. J. (1997). Integrating Sport and Tourism: A Review of Regional Policies in England. *Progress in Tourism and Hospitality Research, 3,* 129–148.

Chapter 5

Conducting Sport Tourism Events: Strategies for Implementation

Questions

1. What human resource strategies are necessary to successfully conduct a sport tourism event?
2. What are the key considerations in managing a sport tourism event's financial resources?
3. What comprises an effective sport tourism event risk management plan?
4. What are the advantages of sponsorship research in developing a sponsorship proposal?

Introduction

Special events such as sport events have become increasingly important for organizers and sponsors to reach their target market. Indeed, we have observed fierce competition to host sport tourism events. In chapter 4, we looked at factors critical to the decision to stage sport tourism events. This chapter focuses on the next stage of transition: key strategies and basic principles for implementation that can be applied to all events. First, administrative strategies concerning personnel and financial and legal matters, as well as risk management will be highlighted. Strategies related to the improvement of community involvement and service quality of event will be reviewed. Various aspects of the operations plan that deal with implementation of the event will be described. These include aspects such as medical services, ticket operations, accreditation, transportation, security, and the like. Public relations and marketing strategies are further highlighted. Finally, attention is paid to wrap-up and evaluation strategies of the sport tourism event.

In Chapter 4, we looked at the organizational structure of the sport tourism event. Attention should also be paid to key administrative functions concerning personnel, financial and legal issues, and risk management.

Personnel and Volunteers

Unsuccessful events often stem from incompetent personnel—a factor briefly mentioned in Chapter 4. Successful events are characterized by effective and efficient use of all resources, including human resources. Most events rely on volunteers in addition to staff to create a successful event. Volunteers may have a strong commitment to the event; however, they may not have the necessary qualifications to perform the job successfully. Therefore, recruiting, training, and maintaining the volunteer workforce are essential.

Determination of personnel and volunteer requirements. Therefore, the first strategy for the implementation of one's human resources will be to determine the number of volunteers and personnel, with the appropriate skills and abilities, required to host the event. Wilkinson (1988) notes that this requires a planned approached whereby one ascertains one's goals and the human resources required to accomplish the plan. Getz (1997) recommends that the program or operational plan be broken down into distinct parts—tasks that people must do to produce the event. A list of the ideal work crew in terms of its numbers, supervisor(s), and skills required should be prepared. The next step will be to determine the current skills and knowledge of those already involved with the event so that one can ascertain additional positions that will need to be filled in order to mange the event (Wilkinson).

Recruitment of personnel and volunteers. Once the personnel requirements have been determined, the recruitment phase will begin. This includes job advertising, shortlisting and recruiting potential candidates, and orienting new staff. With the increasing competition for events, recruitment cannot be left neither to chance nor to the traditional networking that constitutes the basis of most recruitment (Wilkinson, 1988).

As mentioned in Chapter 4, too few events have effective recruiting and training procedures for volunteers despite the fact that they constitute the backbone of most events. Numerous groups and organizations can be contacted for volunteer recruitment. These include community organizations, schools, volunteer bureaus, related government departments, current and retired business professional, and spectators (Wilkinson, 1988). Getz (1997) adds that schools and colleges are an important source of volunteers as internships and projects can be created to involve students in the event. A significant factor in attracting event volunteers may be the extent to which events are discerned to be supporting local community development goals (Williams & Harris, 1988). Targeting specific people known to have desired skills, contacts, or resources is common practice (Getz). In addition, many event organizers ask professionals from diverse backgrounds to be involved in planning and advisory committees. Sponsors can provide a principal source of transitory employment. Therefore, it may be useful to consider making the provision of essential volunteers, or internal recruitment, part of sponsorship arrangements (Getz). Grant-givers, receivers of donations, suppliers, and other stakeholders should also be approached. Depending on the nature of the event, personnel from government departments, school districts, and municipal recreation may also be suitable contacts (Wilkinson).

Volunteers can be recruited on a personal basis (one-on-one or as a group) as well as through various advertising modes, such as public service announcements, bulletin boards, and flyers. Moreover, the event itself can be an influential recruitment medium. A stall with information on how to volunteer can be assembled. Furthermore, potential candidates can be reached by having social events for the community. Information pertaining to potential volunteers, such as name, address, phone number, skills, interests, time availability, and prior experience should be filed.

The selection process may consist of the following elements as outlined by Getz (1997):

1. Applications: Acquire information about the recruit, including abilities, interests, experiences, and references to contact.

2. Screening: Check references; use professional or police security checks for important positions; assess qualifications; short-list the most expedient recruits.

3. Interviews: Use professional recruiters, preferred to avoid bias and ensure precise screening; use prepared and standard questions to allow comparison to come through; personality or skill tests might be helpful.

4. Offers: To avoid misunderstanding, make them in person and in writing; stipulate the job description and working conditions.

5. Negotiations and contracts: Must be done for staff positions, but not common with volunteer positions.

6. Announcements and thank-yous to successful and other candidates.

The key to success in volunteer placement is matching the volunteer with the appropriate job. Therefore, as indicated by Wilkinson (1988), careful attention is required when matching the volunteer's motives to the job requirements. A self-assessment questionnaire can be employed to ascertain the volunteer's motives. As mentioned previously, the next task will be to fit the volunteer to a position that needs to be filled. A brief job description can be constructed in order to furnish a framework of expectations for the volunteer. Getz (1997) notes that it is important to know the steps of preparing ideal job descriptions; however, event managers often have neither the time nor the resources to prepare complex ones. As events become more professional, the job description becomes a critical management tool. In small organizations, one person may be able to perform numerous tasks; in larger organizations, however, job differentiation increases, and workers are more restricted. "Overspecialization," which limits workers to narrowly defined tasks, carries the risk of promoting inflexibility and bureaucracy. For many volunteers, this standard will be neither realistic nor desirable; they will want the comfort of a narrowly defined job description (Getz, 1997). Getz further suggests that the job description should include and identify the following elements:

- Position title

- Responsibility and duties

- Authority

- Tasks

- Key results, performance criteria, and job specifications

- Personal attributes

- Required knowledge and skills

- Commitment

- Resources available

- Rewards or incentives.

It is beneficial to maintain a pool of volunteers who will be available in emergencies and on short notice.

Training of personnel and volunteers. Orientation to the event is a significant aspect of staff and volunteer training. Furthermore, the organization should ensure that its investment is appropriately managed. Orientation should include some of the following aspects:

- Synopsis of the event—basic information about the organization and the event

- Introduction to the central figures, as well as staff and other volunteers

- Introduction to organizational culture, mission, and workstyles

- Report on the significance and roles of volunteers and on policies and procedures for volunteers

- Support available to the volunteer

- Introduction to the training program.

Training attempts to ensure that all recruits and existing personnel can fulfill their responsibilities, grow within the organization, and develop their potential Getz (1997). Getz adds that training may further constitute a reward as many people are seeking new skills. Training is necessary for those beginning responsible positions, and distinct job training may be essential for specific functions. Graham, Goldblatt, and Delpy (1995) suggest that simulation exercises be incorporated into training sessions. Getz notes the following training options:

- Existing staff and volunteers as trainers or more informal mentors

- Team approaches

- Experts for formal sessions and courses

- Conferences

- Professional association programs

- Apprenticeships and internships.

Apprenticeships and internships are unique ways to introduce students to the organization and event management (Getz, 1997). Ongoing professional development for volunteers and staff is encouraged. The effectiveness and efficiency of training should be evaluated, and this evaluation can be attained through systematic performance appraisals (Getz). Getz adds that adequate supervision becomes more appropriate for events that are more complex in order to ensure job performance and satisfaction.

Burnout often occurs as events can engender numerous stressors for personnel because of the intense time and energy commitment inherent to the organization of events. Effective intervention may well solve some of the causes of burnout. Often volunteers feel distressed due to a lack of direction, unchallenging tasks, and feelings of underutilization.

Support and recognition are crucial to developing a sense of belonging and commitment to the event. Uniforms, pins, certificates, free admission, meals and parking, recognition at closing ceremonies, and thank-yous are among the many forms of recognition that can be employed. However, caution is warranted as it is essential not to overdo the material recognition. The genuine reward is the assignment itself. Subtle forms of recognition, such as participation in decision-making, may also be advantageous. In concluding, sport tourism event organizers should take cognizance of the significant role that personnel, and particularly volunteers, play in the continual operation and success of the event.

According to the volunteer management plan for the 8th World Swimming Championships, it is predicted that about 1,500 event staff will be required to manage the event. Recruitment programs will commence from January 1997 through the respective disciplines, parent bodies, and relevant organizations. Preference should be given to experienced staff who assisted with the 1991 6th World Swimming Championships in Perth. Contact addresses, invitations, acknowledgments and employment details will be stored on a database. An extensive training program will be executed to ensure coordinated management, meaningful and varied employment activities and a wide range of ongoing benefits for individuals and associated organizations. Volunteer staff will receive official uniforms, meals during the Championships period, references on request, and access to the final "thank you" party. (Melchert, 1997, pp. 53–54)

Sport Tour: Volunteer Services Subcommittee for the 8th World Swimming Championships, Perth, 1998

Financial Strategies

Financing and budgeting are essential implementation strategies to ensure that the event incurs no loss or, more important, makes a profit. Planning and budgeting are inextricably linked. Getz (1997) contends that budgeting and programming go together, as the program manager may have to fight for a big segment of the financial plan, then appropriate the resources among competing program elements. Furthermore, regarding the organization and hosting of any event, irrespective of size and complexity, "finances" is a bottom-line, basic standard (Wilkinson, 1988).

Sport Tour: Volunteer Services Coordinator—Duty Statements for the 8th World Swimming Championships, Perth 1998

The Volunteer Services Coordinator is responsible for the preparation and implementation of arrangements for volunteer staff for the 8th World Swimming Championships. The Volunteer Services Coordinator will work under the direction of the Volunteer Management Committee and is responsible to the Operations Manager. Specific responsibilities:

- *Coordinate the recruitment process of the volunteers*
- *Oversee the data entry and allocation of volunteers to positions and the interview process*
- *Prepare, issue and manage volunteer rosters and manage volunteer sign/off venue*
- *Coordinate volunteer training and information*
- *Coordinate volunteers uniform supplies and distribution*
- *Coordinate volunteer services i.e. Meals, parking, accreditation, information bulletins, messages, lockers/storage areas*
- *Coordinate volunteer recognition and awards program*
- *Coordinate daily briefing sessions for volunteer*

(Melchert, 1997, p. 32)

The budget for the event consists of the planning of revenue and expense, usually with the goal of achieving a target level of profitability. The budget is often presented in a spreadsheet that shows all activities of the event and the anticipated or planned revenues and expenses (Wilkinson, 1988).

Consideration should be given to the following financial stipulations as outlined by Wilkinson (1988):

• Any activity considered costs money or will necessitate an expense.

• As many events are in the planning stage for many months prior to the actual event, inflation is a factor that should be accounted for.

• The longer the time frame between planning and actual expenditure, the greater the difference between anticipated cost and actual cost. Therefore, a contingency factor is recommended.

• Policies should be in place before a budget is produced. In this way, one can ensure no cost overruns due to a change of policy halfway through the planning of an event.

• Financial considerations should be managed together with planning the event as planning will continuously refocus and emphasize the goals and intentions of the organizing committee.

Cost-Revenue Management

Because many events depend on gate revenues and event-related sales, costs might be controlled but revenues are highly variable. To ensure the financial health of the event organization, *cost-revenue management* is a strategy that can be used to identify and manage all cost and revenue centers (Getz, 1997). Getz notes the following goals of cost-revenue management:

• Secure long-term, anticipated revenue sources that will meet basic organizational costs.

• Tie program components to specific revenue sources such as sponsorships and grants.

• Emphasize revenue-generating activities.

• Control and reduce cost centers (i.e., program or management areas).

• Have other organizations assume responsibility for financial risks or aid with covering shortfalls.

Budgeting, record keeping, and financial control. Budgeting, record keeping, and financial control are three important strategies required to ensure that your financial operation functions effectively. Managers use budgets to predict their financial future, to help set priorities and plan the event, and to keep spending within limits (Getz, 1997). *Operating budgets* are used to plan for one financial year of operations; *capital budgets* are prepared for capital acquisitions; *and cash budgets* are used to summarize planned cash receipts and disbursements (Getz).

In many events, budget procedures have been inadequate. In many instances, this has occurred because event organizers use the previous year's budget and only adjust for inflation. This approach is known as *incremental budgeting.* Managers prefer to build and look for growth and improvements; however, they assume that last year's budget was perfect. In order to prevent this from occurring, many corporations have turned *to zero-based budgeting* (Z.B.B.). By this process, each manager must justify the entire budget request from scratch; therefore, previous budgets are excluded. Wilkinson (1988) further adds that in Z.B.B., the organization's goals are the major criteria for assigning resources, and all activities are evaluated and prioritized. Similarly, Pike Masteralexis, Barr, and Hums (1998) assert that this form of budget process compels event managers to view their event from a new perspective, thereby assisting them in seeking ways to become more effective and efficient. Z.B.B. is one type of budgeting that is recommended. It provides a practical method regarding why one spends and what one spends, and it is particularly useful during an event when revenues are oscillating and quick budgetary judgments are required. Moreover, it is more closely tied to the annual evaluation process whereby success must be verified and not presumed (Getz, 1997).

Getz further suggests that budgets be discussed and debated as they set financial goals as well as spending limits. For example, the budget will allocate projected revenue among possible competing functional area managers, thereby determining the activities for the coming year. The budget will also prioritize elements of the event program.

Precise record keeping and financial control of all funds coming into and being spent by the event is critical. Bookkeeping is the foundation for adhering to sound accounting practices. Two forms of bookkeeping are common in event management, namely, cash-based accounting and accrual-based accounting. In the cash-based accounting method, transactions are accounted for only when cash changes hands. The principal intent for using this method is that one does not spend what one does not have. Accrual-based accounting records transactions when expenses are incurred or income is appropriated. This approach is often required when there are considerable unpaid bills in any reporting interval. Thus, to display a true picture of the financial status of an event, the accrual method is often preferred over the cash-based accounting system (Wilkinson, 1988).

Wilkinson further reports that many successful events have been recorded with joint use of both methods. In such cases, the books are maintained on a cash basis, but during each reporting interval, the necessary adjustments are made to record the accruals for statement purposes.

The fundamental constituents of a bookkeeping plan necessitate recording, classifying, and summarizing financial transactions so that information can be utilized by managers and accessible for external auditing. Financial reporting consists of the preparation, presentation, and ratification of an event's financial status (Wilkinson, 1988). Budgeting and recording are, therefore, two essential strategies, as well as primary ethical and legal requirements, for success. Managers should ensure that the agreed-upon budget is adhered to, that money and resources are used only with proper authorization, and that revenues are secure and properly recorded. Financial controls are thus required for cash, inventory, reimbursements, credit, and ticketing. The nature and scope of the event will determine the number and skill levels of an events financial professionals and volunteers.

Cash-Flow management strategies. To adhere to the budget and to have a tool for setting and revising budgets, the sport tourism event manager must be able to regulate and predict cash flow. The basis of cash flow is to precisely forecast all expenditures and revenues for every month of the budgetary period (Getz, 1997). For many events, costs are ongoing, and revenues generally come from the event at the end of the budget year. Getz (1997) recommends the creation of a cash-flow "calendar" showing the times at which expenditures must be made and revenue is to be realized. In using such a calendar, potential shortfalls are identified. Shortfalls are not inevitably catastrophic; however, the event manager must have a strategy for dealing with them. For example, suppliers can be persuaded to delay their bills until the end of the event, or sponsors can be approached to advance some money.

Legal Issues and Considerations for Implementation

A number of important issues from the perspective of an organizer of an event are highlighted in this section. It is geared towards gaining a working knowledge of relevant legal issues as applicable laws will vary depending upon the jurisdiction. It is important to note that these factors are not comprehensive and may vary depending upon the nature of the event. In most instances, it will be the organizer's duty to arrange for a venue for the event, and many of the other contracts for the event will be subject to this arrangement.

Venue contracts. Contracts for venue are usually in the form of a license or lease. Levine (1987) asserts that whether it is a lease or a license agreement, the agreements must clearly set forth factors that include some of the following:

1. Parts of the facility that will be accessible for the event

2. Exact times when the facility will be available, including preparation

3. Amount and terms of payment

4. Stipulation of use of stadium, arena, fields, and/or other facilities

5. Accountability for all setup work and post-event cleanup

6. Venue insurance

7. Access to venue signage

8. Permits required from the appropriate agencies (a city council, for example, in the case of a motor rally).

Negotiations regarding covering up existing signage may be required, or existing contracts should be renegotiated. A variance contract may be applied for; it suspends all other agreements for a specific period of time while the sport event tenant occupies the venue.

Sponsorship contracts. With regard to contracts for potential sponsors, the primary concern for sponsors is associating their name with the event, and all that it entails. Levine (1988) maintains that in a typical contract between an event organizer and a sponsor, the following issues require consideration:

1. Specific dates of event

2. Exclusive right to associate name of sponsor's choice with the event

3. Exclusivity for the main sponsor (The organizer may want to retain rights to secure additional sponsors who do not compete in same marketplace as main sponsor.)

4. Trademark/registered user agreement

5. Complimentary tickets and/or boxes arranged for sponsors

6. Stipulations regarding appropriate signage and cost of signs.

The most important item in contracts between sponsors and event organizers is exclusivity—the exclusive sponsorship rights per product category or service (Graham et al., 1995). Graham et al. recommend the following "exclusivity plan":

1. Determine which rights require exclusivity and list them in order of priority of value to your organization and the event as a whole.

2. Identify the rights that are negotiable.

3. Assign a value and negotiating range to each item that unconditionally requires exclusivity.

4. Use qualified sport event legal counsel to assist with the contracts governing exclusivity.

5. Distribute exclusivity agreements to critical parties, and request their remarks before concluding negotiations.

Sports-governing bodies. In the case of sport tourism events, it is possible that the organizer will have to contract directly with a sports association in order to obtain rights to an event. Each sports body will have its own particular rules and regulations that must strictly be observed.

Media coverage and promotional rights. If the event is of sufficient size, the organizer will be able to sell the rights to broadcast the event on TV or radio. The organizer, therefore, will enter a license agreement with the broadcaster granting the right to broadcast the event for a set license fee. It is recommended that the organizer retain some advertising time on the broadcast for itself and sponsors of the event.

Liability to spectators and participants. Although the organizer does not have to protect the spectator or participant from every conceivable risk, reasonable care must be exercised to protect a spectator from the most serious cases. Spectators may also be harmed by the action of other spectators. Generally, the organizer is not accountable for the independent actions of spectators but will be liable if there has been insufficient supervision, particularly if clamorous behavior is being tolerated (Levine, 1988). Participants may be injured in the course of the event as well. It is generally understood that risk is associated with the roles they assume. The organizer should further be prepared to deal with emergency medical or security problems that may arise in a large public gathering.

Political contingencies. With regard to sponsorship agreements, it is recommended that the parties contemplate clauses regarding termination of the agreement in the event legislation is passed restricting or prohibiting the sponsor's ability to promote or advertise its products in association with the event (Levine, 1988). Tobacco sponsorship is a case in point because legislation prohibiting its promotion and advertisement is continuously being considered.

Insurance. It is evident that an organizer of a sport tourism event will be exposed to numerous potential liabilities. Therefore, it is imperative that the organizer accurately assess such risks, take measures to prevent them from occurring, and establish adequate insurance coverage to be protected from such risks (Levine, 1988). The insurance contract will shift some or all of the risk of potential liabilities to the insurance company. More than likely, the sport tourism event organizer will require that the venue owner have a minimum level of insurance. Examples of typical insurance coverage for an event include general liability insurance, performer medical insurance, cancellation insurance, television mechanical breakdown insurance, and worker's compensation (Graham et al., 1995). The premium for these forms of insurance will be based on the level of risk associated with the event. As the different types and forms of insurance policies are so diverse, it is recommended that the organizing committee contact an insurance agent who is knowledgeable in this domain.

Risk Management

In order to reduce the risk of accidents and injuries arising, the organizer is morally obliged to organize and manage the event in the safest possible way. *Risk management* can be defined as the process of anticipating, preventing, or minimizing potential costs, losses or problems for the event, organization, partners, and guests. Berlonghi (1990) notes that risk management is becoming increasingly essential for the success and survival of any event.

Getz (1997) contends that the following factors should be considered as they present risks unique to events. Large crowds by themselves are not problematic. However, if they are combined with management and site deficiencies, they can be potentially disastrous. Moreover, the bigger the event, the more likely it will be targeted by protesters, criminals, and terrorists. Events that allow alcohol consumption require an alcohol risk management system. Some target markets, for example, tourists from different cultures, may pose certain risks. Iranian diplomats were concerned about the treatment their citizens would receive at the 1996 Summer Olympic Games in Atlanta because of the previous military hostilities between Iran and the United States..

Two approaches identified as critical to the management of risks associated with an event are the development and implementation of a risk management plan and the purchase of appropriate insurance coverage (Pike Masteralexis et al., 1998). Levine (1988) identified a framework for comprehensive risk management that includes the following:

1. Identify all areas of potential risk (risk analysis).

2. Exclude or reduce risk by arranging education/training programs, safety programs, and inspection procedures.

3. Establish protective funds to cover risks that cannot be eliminated or presumed.

4. Expand technical assets to carry out risk management plans.

Berlonghi (1990) suggests the following generic risk management strategies:

1. Avoidance: Pursue methods to anticipate, avoid or reduce risks. If the risk is too great, avoid it by elimination. For example, the swim portion of a triathlon may be cancelled if race organizers deem the water too cold or unsanitary for participation.

2. Reduction of hazards: Minimize some hazards through better management, training, or operations.

3. Reduction of severity of damages and losses: As problems do arise, have emergency response procedures and contingency plans available.

4. Diffusion: Consider spreading risks among stakeholder or over space and time. For example, vendors and suppliers can provide their own insurance, thereby sharing in the risk management process.

5. Reallocation: Completely reallocate risks, for example, when a municipality absorbs risks for specific events.

6. Insurance: As discussed previously, have the coverage necessary to protect against risks that materialize.

It is important to note that although sport tourism event managers can implement a number of risk management strategies, doing so does not exonerate them from all responsibility and liability concerning the event. These managers are nevertheless responsible for organizing an event in a responsible, safe manner, or they may be found liable for any injuries or problems that may arise (Pike Masteralexis et al., 1998). Pike Masteralexis et al. conclude that sport tourism event organizers should recognize the significance of addressing risk management concerns associated with an event in order to confine the legal liability of the event.

Community Involvement Strategies

The importance and prestige associated with major sport tourism events often lead to fast-track planning practices that ignore community resistance to hosting the event or the construction of associated infrastructure (Roche, 1991). Hall (1989) recommends community involvement as it encourages local flavor in the nature of the event and the tourist destination, assists in the protection of the tourist resource, and reduces opposition to tourist development. Events are tourism products that cannot be forced onto the host community if the community opposes such events. Moreover, by using consultative measures that encourage residents to assist in the planning of and for the event, residents may come to feel that they own the event. Consequently, it may become a source of community pride that may further encourage appropriate tourism development (Hall, 1992). For any sport tourism event to be successful, it is critical to gain the interest and support of the community. In order to maximize the level of community support for an event, an advisory committee may be formed that has a broad representation from throughout the host community (Hall, 1992). It may include members from various groups, such as government, service clubs, educational institutions, unions, cultural associations, and youth groups. Involving the community can assist in building relationships for the future.

Quality Service Strategies

In chapter 6 we look at Zeithaml, Parasuraman, and Berry's (1990) approach to service quality. They argued that service quality could only be defined by considering the customer's experiences, satisfactions, and expectations. It is, therefore, important for event managers to know their audience and consider their target markets before setting quality standards. To ensure that delivery meets the specifications, specifications and performance criteria for each program element and service encounter should be formulated and communicated to all personnel (Getz, 1997). In addition, Getz suggests the following sources may be useful for evaluating the service quality for events:

- Customer reports on satisfaction, complaints, likes, and dislikes

- Peer evaluations of staff and volunteers

- Self-reporting by staff and volunteers

- Objective measures of conformity to service procedures (by supervisors)

- Objective measures of defects and problems and the number resolved effectively

- Subjective measures (e.g., of personal conduct and attitudes)

- Deviation from average, minimum, or delivery and response times.

Service Quality Training

Many elements of service quality are subjective; therefore, staff and volunteers may have difficulty understanding what kinds of behavior are expected, discouraged, or empowered (Getz, 1997). *Critical incident analysis* is a useful training and evaluation tool to increase their understanding of service quality. Bitner, Booms, and Tetreault (1990) identified three groups of incidents in which the service staff reacts to customer complaints or disappointments, responds to customer needs and requests, and takes unsolicited actions related to guests. These behaviors and responses can be observed during real event situations or through role-playing. It is critical that personnel be trained and empowered to use discretion and have a reasonable idea about the limits.

Operations Plan

The operations plan deals with the implementation of the program and venue plans (Getz, 1997). However, operational planning also influences site and programming details; therefore, all these plans should be determined in conjunction with each other. The operations plan translates the program into the reality of the event.

Medical Services Operations

Planning for medical emergencies is an important factor for an event's success. The provision of medical services involves the supply of spectator first aid, participant safety, and emergency services. Medical support staff and external services, such as ambulances and hospitals, should be incorporated into the plan. Personnel could include physicians, physiotherapists, certifies athletic therapists, registered nurses, and emergency medical technicians. Nonmedical personnel can also be trained how to respond appropriately in the case of an emergency. First aid stations, for both participants and spectators, should be set up at the venue. Wilkinson (1988) recommends the formulation of an emergency plan. He adds that this plan will vary depending on the site and activity. Emergency exits should be identified. Furthermore, the closest hospital should be identified and informed of the event.

Communications Operations

Communication for an event is related to every area of the event because all committees and individuals require access to information and to each other. The working mechanics of all aspects of communication to guarantee its success must be defined. The communication requirements for each group should be assessed. Communications provides the fundamental component of information to an event. This information may be furnished in the forms of message boards, walkie-talkies, or internal newsletters. Telephones, faxes, and computer systems may also be required. Irrespective of the level of sophistication, it is crucial to ensure communication with everyone at all times.

Ticket Operations

The ability of an event to charge admission is dependent, to a large extent, on the location of the event and how well the event manager can control entry to the event (Pike Masteralexis et al., 1998). For events that will be charging admission, ticket sales as a means of admission control are necessitated. The first step in the ticket planning process is to consider whether to sell reserve seats or general admission seats. Wilkinson (1988) maintains that smaller events can generally be managed with general admission seating. Likewise when an event is being held in a larger venue, but a capacity crowd is not anticipated, general admission seating can also be used. In some instances, the nature of the event, for example, an open field for a hot air balloon show or a roped-off section behind the home plate area of a baseball tournament, makes general admissions the only practical method of admission. Reserve seating may be the best method of ticketing when a large attendance is expected as people would like to know where they will be seated upon purchasing their tickets (Wilkinson, 1988). Moreover, Getz (1997) recommends events use reserved rather than general admission seating because it prevents the risk of crushes as people attempt to get the best spots. People also tend to become frustrated and tired from waiting in lines. The type of admission and seating plan that is ultimately selected will determine the level of logistical planning required for the event. For example, general admission seating will require more security to direct and contain the spectators.

Ticket pricing. Ticket pricing is the next step to be considered. As Getz (1997) suggests, an event can choose from a range of price structures that include

- Single admission price for everyone, or differential pricing based on age, time, groups, etc.

- Free general admission, but with a price for specific attractions, or admission price plus charges for specific attractions

- Free admission, but charges for extras such as parking, reserved seating, program, etc.

- No charges, but with recommended "donations"

- No charges for those conforming with special prerequisites, such as the wearing of particular costumes

- Sponsor-provided discounts promptly available to offset the price

- Single admission, multi-visit, or season tickets.

One must determine what the public will pay for the event. Even when the economy is booming, almost every event has a point at which the price is no longer elastic and consumers will refuse to buy (Catherwood & Van Kirk, 1992). Consideration should, therefore, be given to pricing at other similar types of events. Local conditions further need to be considered. For example, at the Los Angeles Olympic Games, the tickets for the soccer games were as low as $7 as the United States was not a soccer nation. In offering low-priced admission, the event attracted huge crowds as it became an event for entire families and attracted an abundance of Latino fans from the southern California area. Attention should also be paid to the number of cut-rate tickets sold when establishing prices for the event. For example, children and senior citizens sometimes pay reduced prices, and seats are usually reserved for corporate sponsors, government officials, and the like.

Ticket reporting. Security for ticketing and admissions is essential to ensure the safe collection, accounting, and deposits of funds (Graham et al., 1995). Moreover, ticket reporting is desirable. For small events, written notes and reports will be adequate. For larger events, or annual events, it may be desirable to issue tickets in conjunction with a form for the event ticket seller to prepare that stipulates the number of tickets received, returned, and sold and cash returned.

Facilities and Equipment Operations

The provision of venue(s) and equipment that will be required to operate one's event is a fundamental element in the management of the event. The facility may be an existing course, field, stadium, or pool, or possibly a new venue still to be constructed. The selection of the facility will depend on the requirements of the event. The venue should fulfill all the technical requirements of the activity. It should further provide adequate control for a variety of factors, such as security, parking, sanitation, maintenance, concessions, and storage, amongst others.

The equipment requirements for each committee should be established. Moreover, committee availability before, during, and after the event should be ascertained. Setting up the equipment, making it operational during the event, and returning it afterward will provide a successful strategy to manage an event (Wilkinson, 1988).

Security and Emergency Procedures

Ensuring the safety and security of patrons and participants at an event is becoming an increasingly more important and difficult task. Sufficient preventative measures should be taken to preserve order and to enforce all rules and regulations. Security personnel requirements and the necessary equipment, such as intrusion detection systems and communications equipment, should be ascertained. Security personnel should further undergo an intensive training program in order to prepare them to deal effectively with security issues that may arise.

Crowd management strategies. Crowd management is the facilitation of the lawful and safe experience of individuals within a crowd (Wilkinson, 1988). Similarly, Getz (1997) maintains that crowd management enhances customer satisfaction and the overall event experience. Moreover, he adds that it includes various forms, such as security measures and a number of site design and operational factors. The venue, therefore, has a large role to play in controlling or shaping behavior.

Getz (1997) further contends that an important design factor is the difference in behavior that results from requiring crowds to sit, as opposed to allowing people to stand and move about. He notes that problems can be prevented through a combination of seating and separating fans from different teams/cities, or separating distinct user groups. Attitude and contact of security also contribute to the success of crowd management. The general attitude of security personnel can affect patron behavior and can have enhancing or disastrous effects on spectators' emotions. Good communication with security personnel and patrons assists in effective crowd management. Catherwood and Van Kirk (1992) note that as every event and every crowd differ, it is essential that the organizers know the audience and its psychology if they are going to handle an event without incidents.

Preventative measures to avoid all major incidents should be in place. For example, clear marking of exits is crucial in order to avoid barriers to emergency movement if required. Peak-time congestion is a factor to

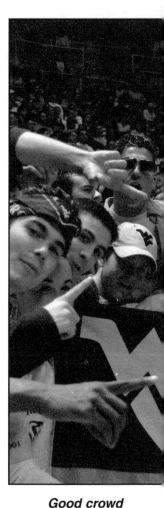

Good crowd management can significantly enhance the quality of a sports event.

Photo reprinted by permission of WVU Photography.

be considered for some events. An attempt should be made to distribute attendance in time or space, or both, through marketing if a site can manage only a specific number at peak times. Another strategy is selling tickets or restricting attendance at gates (through queuing) instead of risking disaster through overcrowding (Getz, 1997). Queuing may further assist in creating a better visitor experience by offering additional entertainment while lining up. However, the number and time length of queuing should be minimized. This can be accomplished by having additional ticket booths.

Therefore, preventative measures as well as plans for managing occurrences that do arise should be in place and known by all security personnel. A crowd management plan that addresses staff training, ejection policy procedures, an effective communication network and the effective use of signage can assist in preventing unruly behavior. Plans should also be in place to deal with issues such as emergency evacuations, hostage taking, bomb threats, and incidents. No matter how small an event, incidents can occur; security and emergency responsibilities should not be avoided.

Alcohol policy. As alcohol is served at many sport tourism events, every crowd management plan should include a comprehensive alcohol policy. Event organizers must be aware of the potential problems that exist with large events as intoxicated persons can cause many problems; resulting in safety concerns to themselves and to others (Farmer, Mulrooney & Ammon, 1996). Berlonghi (1990) asserts that if the sale and consumption of alcohol are managed properly, serious litigation may be prevented. Trained crowd management personnel can be deployed at event facility entrances and prohibit intoxicated individuals from entering. Alcohol consumption can further be controlled by prohibiting patrons from entering the premises with alcoholic beverages. In addition, training individuals who serve alcohol or handle intoxicated patrons is a very significant aspect of a successful alcohol strategy and a crowd management plan (Farmer et al., 1996). Because of the obvious potential for litigation involving alcohol, many facility managers have eliminated alcohol sales. However, others argue that an extensive crowd management plan will assist in reducing irresponsible alcohol-related actions.

Transportation and Parking Operations

The transportation system should be related to the size and complexity of the event. Sound planning of the transportation operations is critical to the success of large and small events alike. Airport, accommodation, and medical transportation planning may be required for larger events. A precise assessment of the number, types, and special requirements of the event participants is important in ascertaining the quantity and types of vehicle transportation required (Wilkinson, 1988). Wilkinson further reports that vehicles may have to be leased; however, there may be opportunities to secure the support of sponsors who may be able to lend suitable vehicles for the duration of the event. This practice is quite common on the Professional Golfer's Association Tour, where automobile dealers lend vehicles to organizers and players, and afterwards, sell them as program or courtesy cars.

Getz (1997) maintains that managers should pay special attention to the requirements of bus tours, the long-distance traveler who is unfamiliar with the setting, and the passing tourist who might be lured to the event. He further contends that traffic operations will be enhanced if tourist and local traffic can be separated.

Routing is an indispensable part of transportation planning, especially scheduled service routes. Operating shuttle buses from parking areas and arranging for special transportation from regional markets will contribute to easing traffic flow (Graham et al.; Getz, 1997). All authorized routes should be clearly marked with signage. Moreover, all signs and information should be positioned for the convenience of the traveler. Travel information should be written and designed for someone who is completely unfamiliar the area. Security routes should further be identified. Assistance in the selection of the most efficient and desirable routes may be obtained from municipal transportation authorities, as well as from police and fire departments. Once a detailed transportation plan has been designed and reviewed, it is recommended that the operations be rehearsed. It is also important to note that factors, such as crowds, unexpected breakdowns and route diversions, may cause totally different conditions during the event. Therefore, Wilkinson (1988) suggests that one build in as many unexpected problems and incidents as possible and test the flexibility and adaptability of the plan.

Permitting pedestrians and normal traffic to mix could be disastrous; Getz (1997), therefore, recommends clear, physical separation of the two. Pedestrians coming to or leaving the site can further create problems, particularly if they arrive or leave at roughly the same time. These situations necessitate police control. Citrine (1995) suggests circular flows for pedestrians within the event site, as such movements reflect natural preferences while avoiding dead ends where congestion can arise. Parades are especially worrisome and necessitate considerable planning with emergency services and detailed police requirements (Getz, 1997). Continual monitoring of transportation patterns is recommended in order to increase or decrease the number of buses required.

Parking management strategies. Parking management is critical for the event's success as it reflects the first contact and impression with spectators, sponsors, and participants (Graham et al., 1995; Wilkinson, 1988). Moreover, as Graham et al. and Wilkinson add, parking generates revenue and may provide goodwill as result of special parking for VIPs and the disabled. Parking is a highly complicated business, and one should plan and implement an efficient and effective parking operation that will provide every vehicle arriving at the site with a convenient parking place. Easy entrance and exit movements of all vehicles and efficient traffic flow in and around parking sites should be guaranteed. The means by which guests, athletes, and spectators arrive should be determined early on (Graham et al., 1995). Different categories of parking should further be identified such as VIP parking, police and emergency vehicle parking, bus parking and vendor and suppliers parking. Consideration to the type of parking system is required, namely, whether parking will be free, paid (cash only), prepaid (a book of tickets) or by means of a pass (allows holder free entry to parking facilities; Wilkinson, 1988).

Concessions and Food Services Operations

Food service should be provided because otherwise famished crowds could go elsewhere and take their food dollars off-site. For small events, one may consider using a volunteer committee or group to conduct and manage all concession operations from buying and preparing the food to selling and cleaning up. For larger events, however, an external company that does all the food services and provides a percentage of the sales or a food service manager to operate the complete concessions/catering program may be more appropriate (Wilkinson, 1988). A food service supervisor will be responsible for handling an endless number of financial and cash procedures; personnel; pricing; and dealing with suppliers concerning contracts, deliveries, and unsold products.

A good operation plan will help and event to profit by meeting the requirements of its customers. It is necessary to consider the type of event, time of event, capacity of venue, number of tickets sold, and weather, especially if food and beverages are to be sold outdoors (Graham et al., 1995). Graham et al. add that service stands should be designed and placed for maximum efficiency and easy spectator access. Besides the food services required by the public, provision should also be made for the participants, volunteers, staff, dignitaries, and special guests.

Sanitation/Refuse Operations

Planning the removal of garbage, restocking paper supplies in the washrooms, and attending to plumbing emergencies are fundamental to the success of the event. All sites to be used should be examined to determine the number and sizes of trashcans required. An inventory of the relevant supplies should be formulated as well as a daily plan for all cleaning tasks and trash removal. In addition to making a daily plan for all cleaning tasks and trash removal, an inventory of the relevant supplies should be taken. The plan should include time and labor required to return the site to its pre-event state.

Accreditation

Accreditation is an identification system that allows access or privileges to those who require access and who must have privileges to fulfill their duties (Wilkinson, 1988). Wilkinson adds that accreditation prevents a condition of total chaos from developing during an event. Its principal benefit is to make the event run as efficiently as possible, permitting the maximum enjoyment by both spectators and participants. Accreditation should, therefore, not be regarded as a policing activity but as a management tool for efficiency and effectiveness in running the event. Accreditation can range from a simple tag for volunteers and personnel to a complex system of computer-encoded credentials with pictures, signatures, and controlled-access security codes built in (Wilkinson, 1988).

The key to success in accreditation includes knowing the participants and all others involved through registration, defining all areas that require information through accreditation, training staff for venue access by ensuring that they understand the accreditation process, and implementing the program with consistency throughout the event (Wilkinson, 1988).

Accommodations

Accommodation planning is an integral part for events that demand overnight or several days' residency. The related accommodation responsibilities are tremendous and can range from inexpensive university residences to more expensive hotels, and even new games villages. Arranging and paying for facilities, planning the correct number of participants, and taking care of their laundry, security, and food requirements increase the responsibility of the accommodation personnel and volunteers (Wilkinson, 1988).

Guests with special needs. Accommodating guests with special needs is an essential requirement. Fleck (1996) notes that the following guidelines regarding site planning and operation principles provided by the American with Disabilities Act should be applied:

1. Provide specific signs and information regarding the special-need services (in larger print and in Braille).

2. Provide special communications devices (e.g., TDD [telephones for the hearing impaired], closed captioning TV and video; audio instead of printed information, with ALS [assisted listening devices]).

3. Remove physical barriers to wheelchairs in order to ensure access to all buildings, activities, and concessions; consider the width of aisles and the necessity for ramps and elevators.

4. Install accessible toilets and rest areas.

5. Add handicapped parking spots with easy access to the site.

The disabled parking plan is especially critical for temporary venues (Graham et al.,1995). Graham et al. note that events planned in temporary venues do not always plan adequately to assign parking for the disabled.

Hospitality. Hospitality ranges from greeting the participants to giving VIPs the royal treatment. It is concerned with satisfying the needs and expectations of all parties involved in the event, including the participants, spectators, media, sponsors, and other guests. Therefore, the hospitality and entertainment provided by the organization contribute to the success of the event. Hospitality suites provide an opportunity for individuals to network while being entertained. It is imperative to ascertain the needs of all those involved in the event and provide ways to meet those needs. Needs and interests can be identified by sending a questionnaire to a random sample of prospective attendees (Graham et al., 1995). Graham et al. further contend that many potential sponsors attend an event a year before they plan to sponsor in order to become familiar with the hospitality opportunities. Therefore, inviting potential sponsors to an event may secure a sponsorship arrangement for the following year.

On-site event hospitality may be offered as an exclusive benefit included in the corporate sponsorship package or marketed to sponsors as an additional revenue stream for the event (Graham et al., 1995). Graham et al. further recommend that when working with exclusive hospitality providers, it is wise to include the right to quality control of the provider in the contract. In so doing, if the level of service is not up to standard, the event manager has the option of requesting reasonable changes.

Novelties, advertising specialties, and souvenirs are a traditional part of many hospitality programs and serve as a reminder of the host and the experience (Graham et al., 1995). Graham et al. add that for the greatest impact, the item should mention or reflect the company or group giving the gift and have a useful life well beyond the event itself.

Event participants further want and seek recognition, appreciation, and thoughtfulness. By developing and preparing an awards/gift program, one can meet the requirements of sponsors, VIPs, organizers and participants (Wilkinson, 1988). Early consideration of what awards are required and how they will be presented will affect the success of the event.

As the media are primarily responsible for the publicity an event receives, meeting their requirements is critical. Members of the media are accustomed to having private meals and accessibility to press rooms where they can complete their work (Pike Masteralexis, et al., 1998).

For the spectators, good hospitality attempts to ensure that they have a pleasant time. Clear signage to direct participants to various elements of event infrastructure and courteous volunteers can assist in an enjoyable experience for spectators. Pike Masteralexis et al. (1998) add that as most events are regular occurrences, the provision of good hospitality is one method of ensuring event loyalty.

Marketing Operations

Public relations and advertising are methods through which the event communicates with its various constituencies and markets. These operations form part of the "communication mix" used to influence the consumer buying process: informing, educating, persuading, and reminding (Getz, 1997). All communications must be coordinated to achieve marketing goals.

Public relations. "Public relations" is defined by Getz (1997) as the actions and communications of the organization that are aimed at fostering awareness, understanding, and positive attitude toward the organization and its operations. Wilkinson (1988) asserts that publicity is a cost-efficient way to get the message to the target market, to sell tickets to an event, or to assist in attaining funding or sponsorship. In the absence of sufficient money to support an adequate advertising program, publicity must be utilized to its fullest potential (Schmader & Jackson, 1997). Getz (1997) cautions that although costs can be kept low, public relations value is not created without planning and effort. Publicity is a tool used to communicate an organization's activities to the public through various channels, which include newspapers, TV, radio, magazines, newsletters and the Internet.

Publicity is furnishing a service to the media. It is meaningful to maintain one-to-one contact with members of the media. Establishing good relationships with the media may go a long way in increasing chances for publicity. However, it is also important to understand the media. Some of the following strategies suggested by Wilkinson (1988) may be useful:

1. Understand the deadlines entailed in newspapers.

2. Understand the deadlines involved in radio and TV.

3. Find out the type of material that interests them.

4. Establish a key media contact person in your organization.

Publicity can be increased by appealing to the interests of the masses with such activities as naming the mascot or designing the logo associated with the event. Key athletes participating in the event can also be used to generate publicity. Schmader and Jackson (1997) maintain that publicity can be increased in distant areas by making the event locally meaningful in the distant centers. For example, publicity can be generated through individualized media releases to outlying areas and calling of participants to participate in your sports festivals. Organizations throughout the market region can be invited to sponsor bus trips to the event for such groups as the elderly and the disabled. Within the event area, the media should be actively involved in the event. Prior to inviting the media to a conference, ensure that a comprehensive mailing list is formulated. Contact community newspapers, television and radio stations as well the daily and weekly newspapers. Many communities compile an events section in their newspapers. A media conference is designed to disseminate hard news to as many media representatives as possible (Wilkinson, 1988). A media kit or a press release covering the announcement you intend to make should be prepared, and copies should be available for distribution. It is vitally important to ensure that persons who are unable to attend receive a copy of the material immediately after the conference is held.

Advertising and advertising media. There are times when it will be necessary to advertise an event in addition to publicizing or promoting it. This, of course, entails a cost. Getz (1997) maintains that that the essence of "advertising" is not just that it usually costs money, but that specific messages are delivered in a predictable, often repetitive manner, usually over mass media. He further asserts that a common error is to advertise indiscriminately without a focused goal-oriented approach, a point referred to in chapter 4. Therefore, target marketing and a comprehensive communications strategy are recommended. Wilkinson (1988) contends that it is not essentially a good idea to extend advertising to all available media. In some communities, the newspaper is the best medium to use, especially because of its ability to reach local and regional audiences with detailed information in a timely fashion. Newspapers with weekly entertainment guides can also be useful. Getting events covered in travel magazines by hosting travel writers is a good way to reach potential tourists (Getz, 1997). In other communities, radio may be a better option for reaching a particular audience. The advantage of radio advertising is that it is better targeted to certain demographic and lifestyle or cultural groups (Catherwood & Van Kirk, 1990; Getz, 1997). Moreover, radio is more useful to generate wide awareness of, and detailed information about, the event before its occurrence. Occasionally getting the message across during a much watched television program may be the best option. However, TV is generally the most expensive method of advertising. Communication via the Internet has become an increasingly popular method of advertising and providing information about one's event.

Wilkinson (1988) asserts that the publicity strategy should include pre-event, event, and post-event activities; photography opportunities and advertising and television potentialities; and followup. Advertising and other communications present considerable scope for creativity, but also for misleading messages (Getz, 1997). Therefore, event organizers have an obligation to adhere to appropriate laws, advertising codes, and consumer protection laws.

Television. Event management includes a clear understanding of the types of television coverage that is at hand and the effective implementation of television coverage when it becomes available (Wilkinson, 1988). Wilkinson further asserts that television is an important consideration as it can assist in increasing public awareness of the event and afford the opportunity to promote the sponsors' and/or suppliers' involvement and contribution to the event.

> ### Sport Tour: Old Mutual Two Oceans Marathon
> *This site is an example of Internet marketing of a sport tourism event, the Old Mutual Two Oceans Marathon held annually in Cape Town, South Africa.*
>
> - *Race information*
> - *Registration*
> - *Confirm entry*
> - *Route Map*
> - *Training Program*
> - *History*
> - *Results*
> - *Runner's Calendar*
> - *Chat Online*
> - *Classifieds*
> - *Notice Board*
> - *Free Email*
> - *Technology*
> - *Accommodation*
>
> *www.twooceansmarathon.org.za*
> *5 February 2000]*

As every TV station is in fierce rivalry with its competitors, sport tourist events can provide fascinating opportunities for footage of a variety of different types of events. Some events, such as the Olympics, create automatic TV interest. However, for lesser events, managers must work hard to develop news angles above and beyond the norm (Catherwood & Van Kirk, 1992). Therefore, potential visual stories will have to be brought to the attention of the media. The TV production crew should be assisted in meeting their specific requirements at the venue and in pre-event, event, and post-event activities.

In order for a sport event to secure direct-rights fees payment from broadcasting affiliates, it must be able to attract large viewing audiences. Few events, including the Olympic Games, Super Bowl, and Wimbledon, are capable of securing direct rights (Pike Masteralexis et al., 1998). Pike Masteralexis et al. add that if an event is unable to secure a direct rights fee payment, there are two alternatives for receiving broadcast time. First, the event promoter can seek a revenue-sharing agreement with the broadcast outlet. For example, the event promoter can offer to cover production costs in exchange for a share of advertising sales revenues (Pike Masteralexis, et al.). If a partnership cannot be arranged, the event promoter can purchase airtime directly from the broadcast outlet. Graham et al. (1995) contend that this is the least attractive strategy as it is the most expensive alternative to the event promoter.

Destination image creation strategies through sport tourism events. Destinations can use imagery of the events to show something tangible of the culture, to convey the impression of variety, and to leave the impression of activity and sophistication (Getz, 1997). Moreover, scenes from sport tourism events can represent family fun, community spirit, or recreational excitement. Authenticity is another important consideration. Sport tourism events can convey the image of a destination that provides access to residents and a look at their way of life. Creation of a destination theme through events is a generic strategy for destinations. In cases where people have a positive image of a destination but it is one of many choices, a sense-of-urgency strategy can be used to attract these visitors. Getz (1997) recommends forceful messages and images to overcome the noise of the marketplace.

Every event "purchase" should be considered an extraordinary experience in the life of a visitor. The image must combine uniqueness and the reward of being there as many events can be watched on television. For recurring events, it is essential to make the circumstances so magnetizing that repeat visits are assured and word-of-mouth promotions will be strong. Therefore, the event itself becomes part of the image-making process. Every event is an indispensable part of the destination region's image enhancement. Therefore, if an event attended by a visitor is a bad experience, it can have negative consequences for the entire region.

Sport tourism event packaging strategies. Getz (1997) asserts that events are themselves packages of activities, venues and experiences that cannot otherwise be enjoyed. The first principle of packaging, therefore, is to link elements that may be difficult for the consumer to acquire or that comprise value-added characteristics. The goals of packaging for events are related both to the event's marketing strategy and the destination (Getz, 1997). Getz mentions the following goals:

• Attract tourists

• Promote the off-season through event packages

- Reach specific yield market segments

- Generate additional revenue and improve the cash flow through advance bookings

- Enhance the event's image

- Encourage visitation outside the peaks (e.g., weekdays)

- Develop partnerships with sponsors, tour companies, etc.

- Combat competitors.

It will be necessary to determine in advance if the aim of the package is to build attendance, generate revenue, expand market share, or boost tourism to the destination (Getz, 1997). The "group tour" provides volume whereas packages purchased by individuals can serve to attract specific segments. Events can form the "core product," the major attraction, of the tour package or can be an added element to give value to other packages. Targeting packages is favored as opposed to offering one or two for general consumption. Packages can be customized through research and cooperation with the tour and hospitality industries. They should include the appropriate elements, such as accommodation, dining, other activities and transportation. Research will, therefore, be required to provide profiles for existing and potential customers, and the package will have to suit each particular segment accordingly. Many events

> ## Sport Tour: World Cup Travel Services for World Cup USA '94
>
> *The organizing committee of World Cup USA (WCOC) formed a division known as the World Cup Travel Services (WCTS) in order to better serve the needs of the international visitor to the World Cup. WCTS was responsible for assigning to authorized tour groups a unique menu of World Cup ingredients, including: 1994 World Cup tickets (including novel team series trips), hotel rooms, access to air transportation via American Airlines (the official airline), Sprint Prepaid Calling Cards (official long-distance telecommunications company), rental cars, and travel insurance and assistance. Scott Parks LeTellier, managing director and chief operating officer of the WCOC, said World Cup USA was extremely happy to be a pioneer in this field as this was a unique approach to tour packaging by major international events. WCTS was novel in that it did not function as a tour packager or operator, the system used by so many previous World Cups. It was an "ingredients" unit that allowed authorized tour operators worldwide, and domestically, to construct packages that suited their customers' needs, which varied from country to country. ("The World Cup," 1993)*

contain elements that will appeal to multiple segments. For example, some events attract the sport as well as the cultural tourist. Caution is required as trying to attract too many different segments can result in user conflicts. It will be helpful for tourist organizations and convention bureaus to assist or market the packages. Another option will be to work with tour companies to encourage and help them create and sell packages featuring the event.

Sponsorship Strategies

In Chapter 7, sport sponsorship will be discussed as a revenue source for financing sport tourism. The International Events Group (IEG, 1995) defines sponsorship as a cash or in-kind fee, or both, paid to a property (such as an event) in return for access to the exploitable commercial potential associated with that property. IEG adds that sponsorship has emerged as the fourth arm of marketing, together with advertising, public relations, and sales promotion. An event provides the organization with a quantity of products that can be offered to a business, government, or social group to sponsor (Wilkinson, 1988). By presenting sponsors a product that may help them meet their communications requirements, sponsors will in turn provide the event manager with product, money, or exposure to assist in meeting the event requirements.

The Benefits of Sponsorship

The benefits of sponsorship to the organization include the availability of resources that otherwise would not have been available (Getz, 1997). For example, it has boosted professionalism by allowing the retention of staff and the development of management systems. Sponsorship further attenuates the marketing reach through the expansion of their investment, as additional advertising and public relations endeavors are undertaken (Getz, 1997).

In order to attract significant sponsorship revenue, the event manager has to understand the benefits to potential sponsors. Meenaghan (1994) asserts that sponsorship has the capacity, possibly not enjoyed by other methods of marketing communications, to extend to all major corporate publics in a single campaign. It is important to note that small events are more likely to operate in a different environment than that of events in larger cities that deal with major corporations (Getz, 1997). Furthermore, Mount and Niro (1995) contend that local business in small communities may be just as motivated by civic duty as by marketing and that promotional goals can be secondary to goodwill. Therefore, compatibility between event goals and dominant local values may be an important factor in small communities where potential sponsors are motivated by a desire to create a positive community image (Getz, 1997).

Importance of Sponsorship Research

With many events competing for sponsorship, the cost of research, preparing proposals, administering contracts, and serving sponsors can be substantial. Moreover, corporations are aware that not all their customers are sport fans and, therefore, have diverted their spending to music and the arts (Catherwood & Kirk, 1992). Researching and targeting sponsors is probably the most overlooked and undervalued step in the sponsorship solicitation process (Schmader & Jackson, 1997). Risks are also associated with sponsorship such as the goals of the organization being displaced by those of major sponsors. Getz (1997) recommends that event managers have a sponsorship plan and be skilled in managing the process in order to prevent risks. Furthermore, organizers will be increasingly asked to provide a defense against ambush marketing. Another risk is alienation to potential consumers through inappropriate sponsorship, such as tobacco and alcohol sponsorships. Several large-scale events tend to contract out their sponsorship sales and promotional responsibilities to consultants and/or private sector agencies in order to reduce the risks associated with insufficient expertise or personnel selling sponsorships.

The "fit" between events and sponsors is an important consideration. Getz (1997) contends that the best sponsors are not only those that provide the most resources but also those that ensure a close fit between the goals, programs, and images of each. For example, tobacco and alcohol products generally are not suitable for youth sports, health themes, and events wanting a "clean, family" image.

Many events start with small sponsors in their own communities, many of whom feel obligated to assist (Getz, 1997). Getz further asserts that building a firm base of local sponsors is a good strategy. Organizers can also leverage a major sponsorship because obtaining one or more key sponsors will act as a magnet for others (Getz, 1997).

Sponsorship Platforms

Events should be viewed and managed as marketable products in order to succeed at sponsorship (Getz, 1997). Management should

Sport Tour: Buffed Bods, Big Crowds Spell Bonanza for Beach Volleyball

Spreading beyond Southern California—the cradle of volleyball civilization—to points as far east as New England and Florida, two-person beach volleyball is more than a party, it's a phenomenon. No beach? No problem! On this Saturday afternoon, 2,200 tons of sand trucked in from a local quarry have created a beige oasis within the Mesa Amphitheater, 15 miles east of Phoenix. As they say in the Pacific Palisades, California, the sacred ground of beach volleyball, the crowds are stoked. And with $100,000 in prize money up for grabs, including $20,000 for the winning team, so are the players. In the 1970s players used to compete for a handshake and a six pack in tiny beach enclaves north and south of Los Angeles. In 1995, between February and September, male players competed in 29 tournaments across the United States. An unaffiliated women's tour is holding 15 meets in many of the same cities but for a fraction of the prize money. Beach volleyball made its debut as a medal event at the Atlanta Olympics. It has come a long way, and suddenly everybody wants a piece of the lifestyle.

Things began to change in the late 1970s and early 1980s, when marketers Jose Cuervo tequila and the Miller Brewing Company saw a potential profit spike in the sport's combination of barechested hedonism and fierce competition. They began offering tournament prizes upward of $10,000 in exchange for conspicuous display of their logos at tournaments along the California coast. By 1983 there were 13 venues. During the 1995 season, Nestea, PowerAde, and Coppertone logos proliferated courtside, while players sport personal sponsors on shorts, shirts, visors and even the skin (thanks to removable tattoos). In 1986 TV caught the wave. In 1995 all 29 of the men's tournaments, plus 14 of the women's, were telecast by NBC, CBS, Prime or ESPN (Pitzer, 1995).

therefore increase sales by maximizing benefits to sponsors. Sponsorship is a form of communication that aids in amplifying and aiming the sponsor's message. Getz (1997) suggests that sponsorship has three dimensions:

1. The sponsor's focus: the company, a product, or a brand

2. The strategic and tactical advantages for which the company can use sponsorship

3. The sponsorship platform that entails the choice of event/competition, or sport.

The "platforms" consist of one or more bases upon which sponsors can build on-site plus "augmented" programs. The usual platforms are the entire event and subcomponents; however, the organization itself can be a platform, especially if it produces more than one event. Getz (1997) recommends that event managers systematically audit their organization and event(s) to identify and value platforms and potential benefits to offer, then target them either to general types of sponsors or to specific companies. This will aid in ranking platforms and "offers" in order of value to the key targets.

Many events use a basic hierarchical approach to sponsorship, each with fees and benefits differentiated (Getz, 1997). In doing so, potential sponsors will know how many sponsors there are in each major category, the cost, and associated benefits.

What is the sponsorship worth? There are no magic numbers to assist managers in pricing the event's sponsorship products (Getz, 1997). However, the more successful the event in meeting sponsors' goals the more that can be received in exchange. The balance between cash and in-kind fees should further be considered, together with the competitive situation.

Research into what the competition is doing, who their sponsors are, and what benefits they offer is useful. Sponsors will be interested in the competitive advantage an event offers, compared to that offered by other events and marketing opportunities. This should emerge from the event manager's research as well as through creative brainstorming by the event manager's team (Getz, 1997). Please refer to chapter 7 for additional coverage of this topic.

Understanding sponsors' decision-making. The quality of the proposal was considered important; reflecting on the professionalism of the applicant and past performance of the event is a critical factor (Weppler & McCarville, 1995). Moreover, applicants must understand where and by whom decisions are made in the organization. For example, rejections or delays may occur if sponsorship proposals were directed at local instead of regional or national headquarters. Getz (1997) suggests that strong corporate relationships should be expanded on a continual basis as personal contacts are crucial. Economic impact data, especially from a credible source, add to the credibility of the event itself (Peterson & Crayton, 1995).

The Sponsorship Proposal

A concise, but thorough and attractive, proposal document should be customized for every important sponsorship target (Getz, 1997). Getz adds that the proposal should fit the sponsor's requirements when targeting top companies. Similarly, Graham et al. (1995) suggest that one should ensure that the sponsorship guidelines are requested from respective companies. A good proposal will consist of the following elements:

- Introductory letter listing the key benefits of interest to the company and what is being requested from them

- Details of the platforms and benefits; sponsorship categories

- Background material about the event and its organization: origins, purpose, goals; key people involved with the event; program, photos, press releases; data on visitors, impacts, media coverage

- Endorsements from satisfied sponsors, list of committed sponsors and partners

- Business card for easy reference

Logos, Graphics, Design, and Signage Program

Every event, large or small, has a specific "look" and a specific "feel." The look may vary from a range of colors, symbols, banners, flags, and logos to a complete lack of color or extraneous support of banners, flags, and symbols (Wilkinson, 1988). Wilkinson adds that the feel may be highly competitive or recreational or very structured or relaxed. Many events are discovering that a look assists in attracting spectators and sponsors to their venue.

To design a look for one's event, one must choose the right elements for the design, how to have those elements designed, made, and distributed during the event. The graphics design program can be very simple with one logo or a complex myriad of symbols for each site, event, sponsor, and operational element (Wilkinson, 1988). The essential consideration is the message that one wants conveyed through the look of the event.

Signage consists of the provision of signs at an event that assist in a number of tasks, including providing directions, giving sponsors exposure, and displaying information (Wilkinson, 1988). Wilkinson further maintains that the signage program should accomplish the smooth and free movement of pedestrians, spectators, participants, staff and all vehicles into, around, and out of the site of the event. It should further provide easily seen but unobtrusive instructions and information for all users of the event. Finally, it should offer an appealing display of messages that can be easily and inexpensively manufactured, assembled, and dismantled (Wilkinson, 1988).

Wrap-Up and Evaluation Strategies

A thorough wrap-up and evaluation of the event is an often disregarded and seldom planned for administrative task. Catherwood and Van Kirk (1992) recommend the following shutdown steps to be handled by the event organizers:

1. Security to facilitate departure of spectators.

2. Parking and transportation staff to expedite the flow of traffic away from the venue. Towing capabilities and police traffic control should be considered.

3. Briefing of venue personnel to determine the necessity for followup and to ascertain their recommendations for future events.

4. Processing of payments for various workers such as the cleaning crew.

5. Clean-up crews to remove trash and clean the venue.

6. Teardown of construction assets and/or equipment that were put in place. This may also require reconstruction for the next event.

7. Final accounting processes with various parties.

8. Contract sign-off by venue management as to the satisfactory completion of each party's obligations.

9. Accountability and custody of all the equipment that does not belong to the venue. Such equipment must be returned to the rightful owners.

Catherwood and Van Kirk add that each of these steps will vary depending on the venue and the complexity of the event. As the final stages of shutdown approach, some final communication with the media is recommended, especially if the event was successful and the promoter is thinking of staging another event in the future (Catherwood & Van Kirk).

Getz (1997) maintains that evaluation is a way to constantly learn more about the organization's environment, the intended and unintended outcomes of the event, and ways in which to improve management. Similarly, Wilkinson (1988) contends that evaluation is especially important to the long-term growth and success of the event. An evaluation will further satisfy sponsors and authorities in providing accountability. The purpose of an evaluation, as outlined by the Wilkinson (1988), includes the following:

1. Evaluation of the worth of the event, to clarify use of resources

2. To learn from mistakes and recognize successes

3. To generate support for a future event

4. To improve the management of future events.

Getz (1997) asserts that the most unusual aspect of event evaluation is the complexity of addressing all the perspectives on events; even the smallest events have to consider their impact on the community and environment. Evaluation is, therefore, not something to be added to the event but is an integral part of the planning process. Similarly, Hall (1992) indicates that the cost of evaluation should be built into any event budget and should not be regarded as an afterthought to event management. Wilkinson (1988) maintains that, early in the organization of the event, it is helpful to select certain individuals to be responsible for this area. Getz (1997) adds that in order to maximize the effectiveness of all evaluations, the entire process should be firmly institutionalized. He further recommends that events start out with modest evaluation exercises and work slowly toward more complicated research and evaluation. Observational research is a major component of the evaluation process. At a minimum, a benchmark visitor survey and impact should be conducted and updated periodically (Getz, 1997).

Summary

To conduct a successful sport tourism event, a number of strategies can be implemented. Administrative strategies include the adequate recruitment and training of personnel and volunteers. Implementing strategies such as cost-revenue management, budgeting, cash-flow management, and tight financial control can prevent financial losses. A working knowledge of legal issues relevant to sport tourism event organization is required.

Events present unique risks to an organization; therefore, comprehensive risk-management framework is essential. Gaining the interest and support of the community is an often-neglected aspect of events; it generally occurs as an afterthought. A successful event cannot be implemented without considerable attention to community involvement. Understanding customer's experiences, satisfactions, and expectations is a critical factor in enhancing quality service. Personnel should receive adequate training in order to increase their understanding of service quality. The operations plan is directly responsible for the implementation of the plans. Careful consideration to a myriad of operational functions is required to enhance the sport tourists' event experience. Wrap-up and evaluation procedures are often neglected aspects of conducting an event. They are essential to the long-term growth and success of the event. Conducting a sport tourist event is extremely exciting; however, inadequate management and organization of the event can spell disaster for tourism in that particular region. Therefore, strategies for implementation to deal with all aspects of the event are critical.

| **Discussion Assignments** | 1. Select an event to be hosted in your community and devise a volunteer management plan based upon the requirements of the event. |

2. Review an annual event held in your community and based on ZBB budgeting, identify ways in which cost-revenue management can be improved upon for the following year.

3. Select an event to be hosted in your community and create a risk-management plan based upon the requirements of the event.

4. Review an event held in your community and identify ways in which service quality and hospitality can be improved.

5. Identify an event that you would like to organize and devise an appropriate sponsorship proposal for selected sponsorship targets.

Chapter 6

Evaluating Sport Tourism

Questions

1. Why do sport tourism organizations evaluate their operations?
2. What are some of the ways in which sport tourism marketers evaluate their sponsorships?
3. What are some of the issues in conducting sport tourism evaluation?

Introduction

There are several reasons why sport tourism event organizers evaluate their services. To better serve customers in the future, those with a true marketing philosophy and concern with customer satisfaction and service quality want to know how consumers perceive various elements of their event (e.g., cleanliness of spectator viewing areas, access for people with disabilities, food concession quality or variety). Many event marketers also develop profiles of consumers in order to target event promotions and sponsorship arrangements toward a desired audience. Some event organizers conduct research to demonstrate to budgetary decision-makers the importance of the event to the host community in effort to maintain or gain future financial resources from the public.

The body of literature on sport event evaluation is voluminous and distinct, with four themes or tracts emerging as important and timely to managers:

(a) customer satisfaction research,

(b) sponsorship evaluations,

(c) economic impact assessments, and

(d) host perceptions of event impacts.

These themes form the major discussion points of this chapter, with the exception of economic impact research, which was discussed in Chapter 2.

Tourist satisfaction is critical to the success of any sporting event, yet relatively little research has been published on this topic in the field's leading journals. Cunningham and Taylor (1995) state that more advances have been made in producing higher quality and more marketable events than on the manner in which the events affect the guests. They further underscore the importance of marketer's knowing what guests think about their event experiences:

> . . . understanding how events affect consumers will help event managers and corporate sponsors design more effective event marketing programs to accomplish specific, consumer-related objectives. Once greater understanding about consumer behavior has been achieved, then more meaningful measures of event marketing effectiveness can be developed (p. 128)

Sport Tourist Satisfaction

Examples of customer satisfaction research applied to sport tourism events include the Elaboration Likelihood Model of Persuasion, which measures guests' involvement with the products associated with the event; heuristics, which explores personal decision-making rules used by the guest to help simplify the decision-making process when dealing with the information in advertisements; and celebrity endorsements, in which guests transfer their feelings about the celebrity endorser to the event and the products sponsoring the event).

In 1995, North American businesses spent $4.7 billion on sponsorship with more than $3 billion on sport. The remainder of sponsorship dollars went to pop music and entertainment tours, festivals, fairs, annual events, the arts and causes. The highly competitive nature sport event production has lead more businesses to demand that event organizers demonstrate the value or return on investment resulting from the sponsorship. This places pressure on the sponsors. They can no longer view their sponsorship as one-sided, benefiting only them, but instead must see it as a relationship which creates a win-win situation for all parties involved. (Cunningham & Taylor, 1995)

Sponsorship Evaluation

Until recently, sponsorship effectiveness studies were uncommon. Reasons for this were difficulty in measuring the return on investment, undeveloped measurement techniques, and high cost of research. Sponsorship assessment techniques now include audience research (on-site and mailed surveys, on-site and phone interviews), attitude/image change studies (longitudinal tracking survey instruments), feedback from trade (employee response), market share data (compare effectiveness of marketing strategies to determine which works best), sales data, and measured media coverage (Cunningham & Taylor, 1995).

An 800 telephone number measures effectiveness by calculating how many guests take advantage of its availability. Bonus offers, such as coupons and free demonstrations, measure effectiveness based on the quantity redeemed. The Internet and online are used as survey/interview services, which determine effectiveness depending on the number of people tapping into the service. On-site computer terminals are used in the same manner as the Internet. Two of the most appealing qualities the above research methods possess are their ability to be less intrusive than, for example, phone surveys or one-on-one interviews, and computer-based surveys can be done at the leisure of the consumer. The above mentioned are possible research options for the future, yet they are still in the infancy stage, and further testing needs to be done.

Researchers of large-scale events have measured the effectiveness of promotional efforts through spectator recall and recognition studies. Previous research in this area has focused on the influence of on-site special event advertisements on spectators' awareness of advertisers' products or services. For example, a study on sport event signage revealed that 59% of those surveyed usually noticed sponsor or brand logos at events and 54% had a more favorable attitude toward the companies involved (Friedman, 1990). Johnson (1992) reported that 43.5% of Chicago Blues Festival attendees identified the event's title sponsor, Miller Brewing Co.; 94% had a more positive image about the sponsoring company, and 73% attested that they would be more likely to purchase a product made by a company that sponsored the event. Such information demonstrates to corporate executives that sponsor promotions influence consumer decision-making and may be useful to festival and event managers in securing resources the following year.

Different companies have created various sponsorship evaluation methods. Many of these methods, like the Anheuser-Busch Sports Sponsorship Evaluation, concentrate on post-sponsorship effectiveness. Sprint has implemented a system that includes both a pre- and post-evaluation. This process has been named the Sprint Sponsorship Vision Project. The system rates certain criteria that have been weighted accordingly:

1. Revenue opportunities for the company

2. Ability to integrate the product into the sporting event

3. Costs of the sponsorship

4. Exposure to the company's target market

5. Company image enhancement gained from the sponsorship

6. Company's competitive advantage gained in the market place through the sponsorship

7. Hospitality/entertainment opportunities for the company that are gained through the sponsorship

8. Sponsorship opportunity to show the company's commitment to the community

9. Through this process, sponsorships can be evaluated and ranked in order of perceived effectiveness. Sport marketers need to be aware of the various decision-making criteria in order to effectively create sponsorship proposals (Brooks, 1994).

Irwin and Asimakopoulos (1992) recommended a pre-event evaluation to sport sponsorship management. The six steps included in this model are (a) a review of the corporate marketing plan, (b) the establishment of specific sport sponsorship objectives, (c) the identification and weighing of evaluation criteria, (d) the screening and selection process, (e) the implementation of the selected sponsorship, and (f) the post-event evaluation.

One of the primary concerns of a sponsorship evaluation is to determine whether the sponsorship goals were met. As indicated earlier in the chapter, sport sponsors seek a number of goals or benefits. If a sponsor's goal was to provide hospitality to prospective clients, the evaluation should determine the number of clients served and their satisfaction levels.

What and *how* questions about sponsorship evaluation should be discussed during the sponsorship deal negotiations. Multiple methods of evaluating sponsorship effectiveness are recommended. A comprehensive sponsorship evaluation of the Kodak Albuquerque International Balloon Fiesta included a post-event survey of sponsors to gauge their satisfaction, spectator sponsorship-recall study, media tracking system, and licensed product sales records. Not all events organizations have the resources to conduct such an elaborate evaluation, but an increasing number of sponsors are requiring that their sponsorship realize a return on investment.

Issues in Sport Tourism Evaluation

Large-scale sport tourism events present several methodological challenges for researchers as such events are typically held over several days, involve multiple events and venues, and attract large spectator crowds. Multiple entrance/exit points, concurrent event schedules, the uncertainty of sport competitions, and in some cases, climatic conditions further compound the challenges. Most research on sport tourism events has involved field surveys of spectators and/or participants. Field survey research has been previously conducted on such diverse events as the Olympic Games (Ritchie & Aitken, 1984), Grand Prix automobile races (Burns & Mules, 1989), and hot air balloon championships (Turco, 1997), with the objective of determining spectator market characteristics, event economic impacts, resident attitudes, and event promotional effectiveness.

This section provides an overview of field survey approaches used at large-scale sport tourism events and describes several accompanying methodological issues associated with sampling and data collection. A conceptual framework for a refined survey method is then applied to the 13th Annual Asian Games to illustrate how contaminants to the validity of field research can be addressed.

Overview of Field Survey Approaches

Numerous field survey approaches have been employed in researching sport mega-events, and several will be described in this section, including interviews; diaries; and mail-back, telephone, and self-administered surveys. Table 6.1 reveals the respective advantages and disadvantages for each technique.

Interviews are commonly used in sport mega-event research. One approach used for spectator studies involves an on-site subject intercept

Table 6.1. Summary of Field Survey Techniques Used in Sport Tourism Event Research

Data Collection Technique	Advantages	Disadvantages
Mail-back	Relative low cost	Nonresponse bias Slow, low return Does not allow for interpretation
Exit interview	Allows for interpretation	Labor intensive High refusal rate
On-site Interview	Allows for interpretation	Labor intensive, intrusive
Telephone survey	Allows for interpretation	Labor intensive Telemarketer contamination Long-distance costs
Diaries	Accurate data	High mortality rates
Systematic selection, Self-administered	Low labor intensity	Incentive to complete may be needed Does not allow for reinterpretation Missed questions, incomplete data
Self-selection, self-administered	Lowest labor intensity	Sample bias

and initial screening. Spectators are systematically selected (i.e., every nth patron passing a designated point), and asked qualifying questions. Subjects meeting eligibility requirements are asked whether they would be willing to participate in the survey. If they are agreeable, an interview may be conducted on the spot. For multiday events, researchers may wish to screen subjects to exclude those who had previously participated in the study.

Systematic subject selection minimizes interviewer bias as untrained interviewers have a tendency to approach individuals who appear attractive and/or similar to the interviewers. In cases where few trained field interviewers are available, a self-administered survey may be used. Subjects are selected in accordance with the aforementioned procedures and are asked to complete a questionnaire and return it to a designated collection box. Often an incentive such as a complimentary event program, souvenir, or beverage is offered to those who complete the survey. A public address announcement reminding subjects to complete and return the survey may be used. Some researchers have used the on-site screening process to develop a list of subjects for a phone or mail-back survey administered shortly after the event. The problem with this approach is that as time passes between the initial contact and the survey, respondents will be more apt to underestimate their actual spending.

Telephone interviews facilitate summative sport tourism evaluations and have several advantages. The process allows interviewers to rephrase questions that may not be immediately understood by the subject. Telephone interviews also generate immediate data collection, leading to prompt analysis. The proliferation of telemarketing has turned off many subjects from participating in telephone surveys. The interview may seem too much like a solicitation and prompt high nonresponse rates.

Exit interviews as a field survey approach, particularly at evening events, tend to produce higher nonresponse rates than do entrance or on-site interviews (Turco, 1995). Spectators exiting a sport venue are often more interested in getting to their vehicles and beating traffic out of the parking lot than in stopping to answer a few questions.

A log or diary is occasionally used for spectator expenditure studies or for studies examining visitor trip characteristics. This approach requires subjects to record their activities on and off the event site during their trip. Although this method has the potential to provide the most accurate information in terms of spending behavior, it also has the highest subject dropout or "mortality" rate. Response rates involving expenditure diaries typically range from 5 to 10%. Even when offered incentives, many visitors find the diary too burdensome and simply quit recording their transactions. It has also been suggested that by recording their transactions, subjects have a heightened awareness of their spending and may alter subsequent purchase decisions.

In all approaches to field survey research, researchers must take care to avoid interfering with subjects' leisure experiences. Such interference leads to higher nonresponse and disgruntled sport consumers. Most field researchers encounter subjects who do not wish to participate in their studies. The question is, at what point does their nonresponse compromise the generalizability of the study's findings? Nonrespondents may be different from survey respondents in certain ways. For example, they may have spent less money, stayed fewer days, and/or attended other attractions. For international events, the language used for field surveys may lead to nonresponse among those who are not fluent. In mail-back survey research, a common practice for addressing the issue of nonresponse bias is to randomly select a subsample of nonrespondents and survey them either by telephone or via direct mail. If responses are statistically similar for this subsample as for the original respondents, it may be assumed that the response group is representative of the population, and therefore, the results may be generalized with greater confidence in their accuracy. If the responses differ significantly, such differences, as well as resulting limitations to the study's generalizability, should be described in the final research report. In the field, subjects are more likely to respond to polite, well-trained, well-groomed surveyors who are dressed in uniforms and possess photo identification.

Sampling

There are two types of sampling techniques: probability and nonprobability. Probability sampling allows each unit within a population the chance to be selected. Techniques within this method include random, stratified, cluster, area, and multiphase sampling. Some would argue that the dynamics of sport tourism events do not permit probability sampling. However, probability sampling can be employed at gated events and those with stadium seating.

Nonprobability sampling is based on judgment, meaning that there is no known chance of a unit being selected. As a result, sampling error cannot be calculated, and we cannot generalize with certainty that the results reflect whole populations (Seaton & Bennett, 1998). Three basic approaches to nonprobability sampling will be covered in this section: convenience, purposive, and quota. Subjects are selected based on their availability and access to the researcher when convenience sampling is used. For certain events, it may be necessary to select subjects who are accessible to the researcher or let subjects select themselves—to volunteer to be surveyed. The resulting *convenience sample* usually consists of those people most interested in the subject, and it is probably unrepresentative of all event participants. With *purposive sampling*, subjects are chosen deliberately, by knowing the type of people they are or where they are located. For example, in a study of corporate sponsorship decision-makers, the few individuals involved are identified and approached directly for interview. A *quota sample* relies on the judgment and ability of the field researchers to select subjects according to certain categories such as age, gender, and ethnicity.

For spectator studies, as the size of the sample increases, more precise sample estimates are achieved. Such sample estimates come closer to true population values because they are more likely to represent all of the subgroups in the overall spectator population (Backstrom & Hursh-Cesar, 1981). Besides sample precision, other factors influencing field survey sample size include the extent to which the population is homogeneous, sampling procedures, availability of resources, and number of analysis categories.

Sample Size

Unless the entire population of spectators or participants at the event is surveyed, the results will have some degree of variability or margin of error. Sport mega-events usually have spectator populations over 100,000 and are considered infinitely large. Attendance and spectator population figures are different for multiple-day events and can be difficult to determine. For example, daily attendance figures must be adjusted to account for individuals who attended the event for more than one day. Open-access events also make spectator attendance counting difficult. Some researchers have resorted to aerial reconnaissance photos with field survey data on spectators and event square footage figures to determine attendance at open-access sporting events.

For evaluations using probability sampling, minimum sample sizes of 385 persons will produce results accurate to within ± 5% of the actual reported figure; a sample of 588 yields results ± 4%; 1,000 generates a ± 3% range at the 95% confidence level. Because greater sample sizes often lead to additional time and financial costs, the researcher must decide how much variability she or he is willing to accept in the study. It is recommended that sample sizes in economic impact studies be large enough for a ± 4% to ± 5% tolerated error level (Table 6.2).

Random sampling is possible at large-scale sport tourism events with stadium-style spectator seating. For example, seat numbers may be generated at random and surveys distributed to spectators occupying the selected seats. Another approach would be to weight the random sample proportionate to the number of seats by ticket price. For events with general admission seating, this stratified random sampling approach is not necessary. Researchers studying sport mega-events with multiple sport offerings must be aware that different events attract different spec-

Table 6.2. Sport Tourism Event Sample Sizes and Precision Levels

Event Attendance	Precision Levels			
	±3%	±4%	±5%	±10%
Under 10,000	1,000	588	385	99
20,000	1,053	606	392	100
50,000	1,087	617	397	100
100,000	1,099	621	398	100
Over 100,000	1,111	625	400	100

Source: Yamane, T. (1967). *Elementary sampling theory.* Englewood Cliffs, NJ: Prentice-Hall.

tator markets. For example, the socioeconomic characteristics of yachting spectators may differ from those of people attending soccer or tae kwon do. This form of sample bias may be avoided by stratifying the survey sample by the number and types of events staged in accordance with projected spectator totals.

Survey Location and Scheduling

Distinct spectator markets attend sport mega-events at different days and times, and congregate in certain areas of an event venue. For example, spectators in luxury skybox suites and those in general admission seating typically possess different socioeconomic characteristics. Young adults are more likely to attend late-night sport sessions than are older adults or families with children. It is neither practical nor necessary to sample participants or event spectators during every hour of operation. Selection of location, days, and hours of operation to sample event spectators must control for sampling bias. Instead, a sampling schedule can be established that assures generalization of results to the total population of spectators.

For multiday events with at least 8 hours of operation per day, a recommended survey schedule is to establish time blocks to conduct the survey. These time periods should be weighted by projected attendance and randomly selected from all possible hours of the event. At the Kodak Albuquerque International Balloon Fiesta, for example, approximately 20% of the total event attendance occurs during the first day; therefore, approximately 20% of the total number of surveys are administered during the event's first day. Table 6.3 provides an example of the survey schedule used for the economic impact study of the 1992 ASA Men's Fast Pitch Softball World Championship Tournament.

Table 6.3. Survey Schedule—1992 ASA Men's Fast Pitch Softball World Championship Tournament

Day	Time	Sample Size
Friday, Sept. 11	6:30–9:30 P.M.	60
Saturday, Sept. 12	12:30–3:00 P.M.	60
	6:00–8:30 P.M.	60
Sunday, Sept. 13	12:30–3:00 P.M.	60
Monday, Sept. 14	12:30–3:00 P.M.	50
Thursday, Sept. 17	6:00–8:30 P.M.	50
Friday, Sept. 18	6:30–9:00 P.M.	50
Total		390

Determining Sport Tourist Groups

Most sporting events do not differentiate between resident and nonresident spectators or determine visitor groups. Rather, attendance totals are used to count the number of spectator visits. Profiling sport tourists, however, requires factoring out residents from the subject database. The following formula is used to determine the number of visitor groups:

VG = ATT × V% ÷ VGS ÷ RATT:

Where: VG = Visitor groups

ATT = Event attendance total

V% = Percentage of survey sample who were visitors

VGS = Visitor group size

RATT = Repeat event attendance.

For example, 94% of all spectators attending the 1994 Illinois Girls State High School Basketball Tournament were nonresidents, based upon results of an on-site survey. Visitor groups averaged approximately four persons in size, stayed in the host community an average of 1.5 nights, and attended approximately two sessions (each session consists of two games). A total of 3,113 visitor groups attended the event. The formula for determining visitor groups was as follows:

3,113 = 27,125 × .94 ÷ 4.09 ÷ 2 (VG = ATT × V% ÷ VGS ÷ RATT).

Sport Tour: 13th Asian Games

This section describes a proposed field research study for the 13th Asian Games held December 6–20, 1998, in Thailand. The games involved 43 national organizing committees and over 10,000 athletes and officials. Thirty-six official sports and two demonstration sports involving 377 events were held at three main sport venues. Bangkok's Rajamangala National Stadium (60,000 seating capacity) held the games' opening and closing ceremonies and was the venue for football and track and field. The compound, managed by the Sports Authority of Thailand (SAT), also features an indoor stadium with a 12,000 seating capacity for sepak takraw, a velodrome, and a shooting range. Thammasat University, Rangsit Campus held track and field athletics, swimming, diving, water polo, archery, football, fencing, wushu, judo, handball, wrestling, sepak takraw, table tennis and tae kwon do. The Thammasat University sport complex consists of the Athletes' Village, a main stadium with seating for 20,000, an aquatic center, and gymnasiums were also allocated for badminton, handball, karate, tae kwon do, wushu, basketball, wrestling, judo, table tennis, fencing and sepak takraw. The Muang Thong Thani Sports Complex hosted boxing, gymnastics and weightlifting, volleyball, tennis and swimming. In addition to these three main venues, sports from archery to yachting were played at 23 other sites throughout Thailand.

This research project would seek to determine the event characteristics most important to the satisfaction of spectators and their perceptions of the quality of these service attributes as delivered by the organizers of the 13th Asian Games. Spectators attending the opening and closing ceremonies at Rajamangala National Stadium would be selected at random to participate in the study, in accordance with their numeric seat assignments. A coupon redeemable for a complimentary beverage would be offered to participants as an incentive to complete the survey at the opening ceremony and a commemorative pin, to subjects at the closing ceremony. A total of 385 interviews were to be completed by adult subjects at both the opening and closing ceremonies. The survey instrument was modeled after SERVQUAL to assess the 10 dimensions of service quality (reliability, tangibles, responsiveness, competence, courtesy, credibility, access, communication, security, and understanding of the customer) as identified by Zeithaml, Parasuraman, and Berry (1990). Survey questions also covered spectator residence and selected demographic variables. At least one member of the interview team would be fluent in the official language for a country participating in the games.

Sport Tourism Research: Longitudinal Approaches

Most research on mega-events has been conducted prior to, during or immediately after the event. Two exceptions are the longitudinal studies conducted by Mount and Leroux (1994) and Ritchie and Smith (1991).

Mount and Leroux (1994) conducted a post hoc analysis of the 1988 Winter Olympic Games held in Calgary on the city's business sector. They compared the impacts (as perceived by businesses) of a one-off event (Olympic Games) with a recurring event (Calgary Stampede). Retail businesses were more affected by the recurring event whereas the service sector was most affected by the one-time event. Businesses that benefited greatly from the one-time event ranked the recurring event as most important to their business. The authors concluded that this response reflects the fact that a hallmark event such as the Calgary Stampede brings annual benefits that are expected to continue and, therefore, would be deemed more important than a one-time event.

Ritchie and Smith (1991) addressed the extent to which the hosting of a mega-event results in increased awareness and enhanced image of the host center/region in the international destination marketplace. Using the 1988 Olympic Winter Games held in Calgary as a case study, they found that levels of awareness and knowledge of the host city in Europe and the United States were dramatically raised. They cautioned that this impact on levels of top-of-mind awareness decreases measurably after a short period of time.

Residents' Perceptions of Sport Tourism

Much has been written about tourists, but relatively little about those who stage these attractions or the residents of the community where the event takes place. Relatively few impact studies have specifically examined residents' attitudes toward sport tourism in their community. One study involving residents' attitudes toward the Kodak Albuquerque International Balloon Fiesta revealed that those who benefited economically and/or socially from the event had more positive attitudes than those of residents who did not experience these benefits (Turco, 1994). These findings are consistent with the social exchange theory, which suggests that hosts who receive benefits from sporting events are likely to perceive it positively and be supportive, whereas those who do not receive benefits or who perceive the costs associated with the event outweighing the benefits, are likely to perceive it negatively.

Why do communities and organizations stage sporting events? The answers to this question may surprise you. Mayfield and Crompton (1995) identified eight generic reasons that nonprofit and government entities stage special events:

1. Recreation/socialization

2. Culture/education

3. Tourism

4. Internal revenue generation

5. Natural resources

6. Agriculture

7. External revenue generation

8. Community pride/spirit.

Of the 30 items identified that operationalized the eight domains, "community spirit/pride" and "family" were ranked by respondents as the most important reasons for staging festivals. Wicks and Fesenmaier (1995) found that business owners and managers felt it was most important that the production of the event brought the community together, generated an economic benefit to businesses, and promoted a positive image for the host town.

Large-scale sport tourism events should examine the contributory social impacts on residents and their reactions. Examples of social costs include traffic congestion and crowding, crime, trespassing, disruption in daily schedules, litter, and noise pollution. Without resident and local business support, several sanctions against the event may be imposed by the community including

1. Loss of local support for the organizations and authorities that promote the event

2. Unwillingness to work at the event or in the tourism industry

3. Lack of enthusiasm in promoting the event by word of mouth

4. Hostility to visitors manifested in overcharging, rudeness, and indifference (Crompton & Ap, 1994).

Important factors in avoiding these social problems, while benefiting the host community, are to focus greater time on measuring the needs and expectations of the residents as they relate to the festival or event, communicating with residents, and getting them involved in the planning process.

Promotional Effectiveness Research

One has only to view a large-scale sporting event and count the numerous corporate names and logos appearing on the participants and signs on-site to agree that the use of sponsor visibility in event management is prevalent (Mullin, Hardy, & Sutton, 2000). Sponsorship and advertising signs are major revenue sources for sport operations. Increasing public and target market awareness of the company and its products or services is also a primary objective of corporations engaging in sponsorship (Irwin & Asimakopoulos, 1992). What influence, if any, does this visibility have on spectators' perceptions of sponsoring corporations and on subsequent consumer decisions?

Sport Tour: Kodak Albuquerque International Balloon Fiesta

The 25th Annual Kodak Albuquerque International Balloon Fiesta was the largest ballooning event in the world, attracting 1.3 million spectators, and 950 balloon pilots representing 18 countries and 48 states. The Albuquerque International Balloon Fiesta, Inc. has annually hosted the event on a 77-acre park leased from the City of Albuquerque. The 1995 event featured a musical concert; four mass ascensions; balloon glow; daily balloon competitions; and food, beverage, and souvenir sales. Activities typically began on the Balloon Fiesta grounds at 6:00 A.M. and continued until 12 noon, except for the concert, Special Shapes Rodeo, and balloon glows, which were held in the afternoon or evening. A field survey was conducted to identify selected characteristics of the event spectator market in order to develop distinct spectator profiles.

A questionnaire developed by the researchers with input from key event officials was used to measure visitor demographics, visitor group expenditures both on and off the event site, visitor group size, residency, composition, and length of stay. Spectator interviews were conducted with a systematic sample of spectators at nine neutral locations on the event grounds to avoid biasing results upward in terms of number of spectators who were visitors. Every 11th adult spectator (n=716) was approached by a trained field survey researcher during 7 of the 9 days of the Balloon Fiesta and asked to participate in the survey. Spectators were also asked if they had previously participated in the survey and, if so, were politely dismissed by the interviewer. Interviews were postponed while the balloons were inflating or aloft. The sampling procedures controlled the distribution of the questionnaire to event spectators, avoided personal bias in sample selection and self-selection by attendees, and assured total numbers contacted and high response rates.

Selection of days and hours of operation to sample spectators and daily sample size targets were systematically stratified to match event attendance figures over the preceding 3 years. Two-hour sampling periods were randomly selected from all 540 possible hours of Balloon Fiesta operations. Data were collected and analyzed as group expenditures. Descriptive statistics, chi-square goodness of fit analyses, and univariate analyses of variance (ANOVA) were performed on the data to delineate market segments and identify significant differences in visitor spending behaviors.

Caucasians represented over three fourths of the total spectator base. Other race/ethnic origins represented included Hispanics (15.7%), African-Americans (3.7%), Asian-Americans (2.1%), and Native Americans (1.5%). The average age of a Balloon Fiesta visitor was 41.7 years. Young adults 18–24 years of age represented 9.3% of all visitors. Adults 25 to 39 years represented 34.3% of the visitor base; those 40–54 years comprised 32.6%; individuals 55 years of age and older totaled 19.0%. Females comprised 46.5 percent of all visitors; males totaled 53%.

Three distinct visitor markets emerged from the data analyses: Big Spenders, Penny Pinchers, and Senior Savers. Big Spenders were primarily first-time visitors to the host community; had high family incomes (most earning more than $70,000); were predominately Anglo; traveled as couples; had longer lengths of stay, and had high retail spending as a percent of total spending. Big Spenders were mostly from out of state, with California, European countries, Texas, and Arizona as primary geographic markets. Penny Pinchers reported shorter length of stay, larger group sizes, tended to stay with friends and relatives or were excursionists, and spent 47% less than Big Spenders. Twenty-one percent were Hispanic, and 58% had family incomes under $40,000. Most Penny Pinchers were from New Mexico or Colorado and had previously attended the event. Senior Savers were older Anglo adult couples from the Midwest and northeast regions of the United States who were en route to Texas or Arizona to vacation during the winter months. Senior Savers comprised 9% of the event's spectator base. Senior Savers stayed in recreational vehicles or budget motels and reported spending totals similar to those of Penny Pinchers.

Summary

Numerous field survey techniques have been employed in sport tourism event research, each with advantages and disadvantages. These techniques include diaries, on-site interviews, and mail-back surveys. The future of field survey research in sport tourism will include technologies that will speed data processing. Voice-activated, hand-held microcomputers linked to cellular phone lines will allow field interview data to be collected and analyzed immediately. It must be remembered that a study, no matter how quickly it is completed, is only as accurate as its methods. Research methods should be tailored to the specifics of the event and not be standardized. The purpose of the study, nature of the sport mega-event, time, and human and financial resources of the research organization dictate the most practical data-collection methods. However, care must be taken to design and implement survey research methods that will negate sampling and nonresponse bias, both serious threats to validity.

Chapter 7

Financing Sport Tourism

Questions

1. What are examples of internal and external revenue sources for sport tourism organizations?
2. What are the different types of fees/charges used by sport tourism organizations as revenue streams?
3. What are the various pricing strategies available to sport tourism service providers?
4. What are the steps to secure sport tourism event sponsorships?
5. What are bonds, and how are they used in the sport tourism system?

Introduction

There are several funding options available to sport tourism operations managers. In *Financing Sport*, Howard and Crompton (1995) distinguish revenue sources as those stemming from the operations of the sport enterprise (internal), and those from external entities. Internal sport revenues include those from charged admissions, sale of licensed products and services, and sale of foodservice and souvenir concessions. Revenues from external sources include sponsorships and fund-raising. This chapter will describe these revenue sources as applied to sport tourism.

Sport Tourism Revenue Sources

This section describes common methods of financing sport tourism facilities and services operations. Revenue sources for sport tourism are classified as compulsory resources, earned income, contractual receipts, and financial assistance. An overview of revenue sources for sport tourism organizations is presented in Table 7.1.

For the public sector, tax revenues are commonly used to finance sport tourism operations, with property taxes as the most common compulsory resource. Portions of state income taxes and gross receipts sales taxes are also used, but less often, to finance sport operations. Some communities rely upon local food and beverage taxes as another source of revenue for sport tourism operations.

The use of hotel/motel taxes to finance sport operations is commonsensical to many public administrators because nonresidents are the beneficiaries of the sport tourism services. Many contend, therefore, that visitors should pay their fair share to support the sport operations via lodging taxes. A concern by some business leaders is that the higher lodging rates due to tax increases may make the destination less competitive in comparison to other communities that have bid to host sport championships.

Compulsory Resources

In the United States, states have traditionally relegated the property tax to local governments as their primary means of raising revenue for leisure services. This source of revenue remains prominent within local systems of finance, especially for school districts, special districts, and county governments. In recent years, however, city administrators have come to rely less on the property taxes for financing their total operations.

Those who consider sport to be a private good argue that sport consumers alone receive the benefits from their transactions, and therefore, such consumers should be the only ones to pay for sport services. On the other hand, those who perceive sport as a public good contend that there are direct and indirect benefits to be derived from sport. Indirect benefits may include an enhanced community quality of life, elevated image of the community as a sport destination, diversified community entertainment options, and improved physical health of residents who participate in sport. Those who argue that sport is a public good contend that direct consumers and indirect beneficiaries should financially support sport operations.

Even though property tax is a traditional form of revenue raising, it suffers from some administrative problems. Large discrepancies in property values result from inaccurate local assessments. Property taxes are also costly and inefficient to administer compared to other tax options. Property tax deters improvements and maintenance on property. Some authorities consider the property tax, currently levied and administered, to be regressive (Morgan, 1984). They argue that the poor pay proportionately more than the well-off do, because the poor spend a larger share of their income for housing than do other groups. Furthermore, citizens who do not use sport facilities and services resent having to pay for them via their property tax.

Table 7.1. Sport Tourism Revenue Classifications and Types

A. Compulsory Resources
  1. Taxes
     a. Property
     b. Income
     c. Sales
     d. Hotel/Motel
  2. Special assessments

B. Earned Income
  1. Fees and charges
     a. entrance fees
     b. admission fees
     c. rental fees
     d. user fees
     e. sales charges
     f. licenses/permit fees
     g. special service fees
  2. Investment interest
     a. endowments
     b. trust fund

C. Contractual Receipts
  1. Land leases
  2. Facility rentals
  3. Concessions operations
  4. Lease, concessions
  5. Lease, lease-backs
  6. Sales
     a. lease-backs
     b. advertising
     c. sponsorship
     d. merchandise

D. Financial Assistance
  1. Grants
  2. Entitlements
     a. specific
     b. general
  3. Special appropriations
  4. Current donations
  5. Planned gifts
  6. Bonds
     a. revenue
     b. general obligation

Special taxes. Municipalities and park districts have the ability to levy special taxes for their leisure services delivery operations through state enabling legislation. Turco and Bretting (1991) found that park district, hotel/motel, recreation district, and special recreation levies were the most prevalent types of special taxation utilized to finance park and recreation operations.

The use of alcohol and tobacco tax revenues (a.k.a. "sin" taxes) earmarked for leisure operations offers an interesting moral and philosophical contradiction for the sport administrator. Some argue that monies generated from the sales of these harmful products should not be used to provide programs and facilities that may improve the physical and emotional well-being of others.

Earned Income

Fees and Charges

Seven classifications of fees and charges are applicable to sport tourism operations:

1. *Entrance fees* are charges to enter a large park, botanical garden, zoological garden, or other developed sport area. The areas are usually well defined but are not necessarily enclosed.

2. *Admission fees* are described as charges made to enter a building, structure, or natural chamber.

3. *Rental fees* are payments made for the privilege of exclusive use of tangible property of any kind. Sport tournament producers often rent stadia to host their events.

4. *User fees* are defined as charges made for the use of a facility, participation in an activity, or fares for a controlled ride. Golf course greens fees are an example of a user fee.

5. *Sales revenues* are revenues obtained from the operation of refectories, stores, concessions, restaurants, etc., and from the sale of merchandise or other property.

6. *License and permit fees* are synonymous. A license is a written acknowledgment of consent to do some lawful thing without command, and is usually issued by a division of government. In the United States, boating, hunting, and fishing licenses are required for participation in these sports.

7. *Special service fees* are charges made for supplying extraordinary articles, commodities, activities, or services as an accommodation to the public.

The literature yields six pricing methods used in determining fees for the delivery of sport services:

1. *Marginal cost pricing.* The fee is set at a price equal to providing an additional unit of the service.

2. *Full pricing.* The fee is set at a level that covers a share of the full cost associated with the provision of the service (Crompton, 1981).

3. *Differential pricing.* The fee is set at different levels for different clients (Crompton, 1984).

4. *Traditional pricing.* The fee is a typical amount that has been charged in the past.

5. *Going-rate pricing.* The fee is a reflection of charges other agencies levy for similar types of services. Agencies scrutinize other pricing structures and then pattern their own fees and charges after them.

6. *Equity pricing.* The fee set at a level that is considered fair to both users and non-users (Crompton, 1984). Concepts associated with this pricing model include the ideas that those who benefit from the services pay for them; a tax subsidy for leisure services is justified only if all taxpayers benefit from those services; and users from outside the community are required to pay for leisure services.

Discount Pricing

Discount pricing offers a way to generate untapped revenue from market segments that are not able, for whatever reasons, to pay the full market value for a good or service. By offering some services at a discount, the sport marketer may maximize service use and realize varying levels of revenue from numerous sources (Cato & Crotts, 1993).

A relatively new discount pricing strategy is to build "fences" that allow consumers to logically segment themselves into an appropriate rate category based upon their consumption behavior (e.g., needs, willingness to pay, usage). The airline industry's advance-purchase and Saturday night stay-over requirements are examples of price fencing. "A price fencing strategy affords price-sensitive users lower rates in exchange for decreased flexibility. On the other hand, full-rate customers can use the services at traditionally higher demand times." (Cato & Crotts, 1993, p. 33). McCarville (1993) offers marketers several suggestions for pricing leisure services.

Principle 1: Participants Seek Fairness in Pricing.

Tip #1: Price is considered most appropriate for those activities that clearly benefit only the participant.
Tip #2: Use other providers' prices as a guide when developing new price levels.
Tip #3: If you must increase your prices, do so in small increments on a regular basis.
Tip #4: Tell customers how much it costs to provide the program they are about to enjoy.

Principle 2: Consumers Seek Value.

Tip #1: Focus on benefits to be enjoyed through purchase.
Tip #2: Assign program names that focus on the benefits of participation.
Tip #3: Ensure your clients know how they benefit from paying a fee.
Tip #4: Compare new programs to well-established and valued alternatives.
Tip #5: Tell the world how wonderful you and your staff are.
Tip #6: Stress the convenience element in all your programs.
Tip #7: Offer liberal refund policies to reduce uncertainty.

Principle 3: Consumers Seek Choices.

Tip #1: Always provide price alternatives
Tip #2: Give the consumer choices as to the kind of price to be paid.

Sport Tourism Sponsorship

Sport sponsorship is big business. The International Events Group (2001) reported that North American corporations alone spent over $5.4 billion on sports marketing in 2000. As the popularity of sport sponsorship has increased, so have the number of sponsorship proposals. Some companies are presented with over 100 sport sponsorship proposals annually (Shelton, 1991).

Sponsorship is defined as the provision of resources (fiscal, human, and physical) by an organization directly to an event or activity in exchange for direct association with the event or activity. The organization can then use this direct association to achieve its corporate, marketing, or media objectives (Sandler & Shani, 1989). Sport is the most popular option for sponsors, comprising 67% of all sponsorship dollars. In North America alone, nearly 5,000 companies spent over $5.0 billion on event sponsorship (IEG, 1996). The top three industries in terms of sport sponsorship spending are the beer industry (20%), the nonalcoholic beverage industry (20%), and banks (13%). Beverage companies Anheuser-Bush, Coca-Cola, and Pepsi all spent more than $25 million on sport sponsorship in 1995. Most corporations pay for sponsorships, considered part of the promotional mix within the broader marketing mix, from their advertising budgets.

For some businesses, sport sponsorship has become an effective marketing strategy and an equally effective revenue producer for sport organizations during the last decade. Increased competition has created a need for businesses to find ways to differentiate their products and services from the growing number of advertisers in the market place and to gain more return for their promotional dollars (Oneal, Finch, Hamilton, & Hammonds, 1987). There are many other reasons that businesses decide to sponsor sport:

1. Demonstrate good citizenship

2. Demonstrate interest in the community

3. Generate visibility for products and services

4. Generate favorable media interest and publicity (Wilkinson as cited in Ensor, 1987, p. 40).

Through increased visibility of the company and its products or services via sport sponsorship, many businesses anticipate increased product and service consumption (Turco, 1994).

Some corporations believe that sponsorships are relatively inexpensive compared to other advertising mediums. Sport sponsorships allow businesses to distinguish themselves from the overabundance of advertisers prevalent in other forms of advertising (Oneal et al., 1987). Increasing market competition and rising costs of traditional advertising mediums also have aided in the shift to sport sponsorship. "Advertisers are aiming to get more bang for their marketing bucks by sponsoring an event itself, rather than just buying 30 seconds of air time during a sports show" (Cook, Melcher, & Welling, 1987, p. 48). The shift in advertising from traditional media to sport sponsorship, coupled with the increased number of sponsorship requests, has made it necessary for corporations to develop a sponsorship evaluation process.

Sponsorship Decision-Making

In Canada, Copeland (1991) conducted a study of the exchange between corporate sponsors and sport groups to gain a better understanding of the decision-making process. Corporate exclusivity was the most important decision-making criterion, followed by

1. Increased company/brand awareness

2. Reinforced company/brand image

3. Signage at events

4. Ability to target spectators

5. Increased sales/trial of product/service.

Of the five different forms of marketing, sponsorship was perceived by the businesses surveyed as the least effective of all marketing and promotional tools. Their prevailing attitude was that to be effective, sport sponsorships should be used in conjunction with other advertising media (Copeland, 1991).

McCarville and Copeland (1994) conducted a study to better understand sport sponsorship through exchange theory. The basis of exchange theory is that both parties offer something of value to each other. Thus, both parties achieve their desired results (Blalock & Wilken, 1979). McCarville and Copeland indicated that sports marketers must find rewards that potential sponsors seek but cannot obtain alone. Offering a variety of benefits helps to keep these relationships appealing. They concluded that sport marketers must understand what businesses are seeking in sponsorships.

Sponsorship Benefits

What does sport have to offer a sponsor? Exclusivity is the seller's prime asset, and it should not be sold cheaply to the sponsor. Exclusivity can be shared between title and presenting sponsors, and also by product categories. The sponsor may accrue several benefits from an affiliation with sport (Table 7.2).

Some corporate decision-makers see sport sponsorship as a way to drive sales whereas others only wish to enhance their image. Irwin and Sutton (1994) found that increasing sales and market share has replaced image enhancement as the primary motive for sport sponsorship. They conclude that image is no longer everything in sport sponsorship. By contrast, McCook et al. (1997) found that the main sponsorship criteria sought by corporate decision-makers were, in priority order, signage/visibility, image enhancement, and increased sales. Similarly, Kuzma, Shanklin, and McCally (1993) found that the top three sport sponsorship objectives for Fortune 1000 companies were to increase awareness of company, to improve company image, and to demonstrate community responsibility.

In a study involving college athletics, Stotlar and Kadlecek (1993) conducted a telephone survey of corporations

Table 7.2. Corporate Benefits of Sport Sponsorship

- Media exposure
- Direct media coverage
- Media mentions
- Signage
- Hospitality opportunities
- Product sampling
- Name association/lifestyle identification
- Enhancement of market's awareness/perception of product
- Merchandising opportunities (product sales)
- Affiliation with other sponsors
- Community pride/involvement

involved with the NCAA tournament sponsorship program to identify the reasons corporations buy sport sponsorships. The primary reasons for sponsorship that companies revealed included (a) the benefits of a corporate affiliation with sports, (b) access to intercollegiate athletic events, (c) media exposure through signage within the venue, (d) ticket access to NCAA championship events, and (e) product/service exclusivity within the sporting venue/s. Supplementary reasons included the (a) desire to increase the corporate consumer base, (b) ability to develop tie-in programs, (c) enhancement of the corporate image, and (d) tie-ins with the current advertising campaign.

Sport Sponsorship Steps

There are six steps to sport sponsorship, and each is discussed in this section.

Step 1. Design the sporting event with sponsorship opportunities. The extensions of the sport tourism event or "product" should be designed to meet both internal and external marketing objectives. Internal objectives would be to satisfy the needs of participants and spectators, as well as to cover operating costs. External objectives would be to satisfy the objectives of, or benefits sought by, corporate sponsors. For example, one of the corporate objectives of Kimberly-Clark, manufacturer of Huggies disposable diapers, is to provide target markets with the opportunity to sample its products. The company is so confident in its product quality that they believe once babies put their bottoms in the diaper, parents will realize the absorption and comfort are the best around, and will be brand loyal, thereafter. The Kodak Albuquerque International Balloon Fiesta, considered the largest hot air ballooning event in the world, was searching for a way to satisfy the needs of one of its consumer market niches, parents with young children. Up until 1995, the organizers of this open-air event had relied upon portable toilets to accommodate the natural requirements of its spectators, much to the inconvenience of parents who wanted to change the soiled diapers of their children. A "win-win" sponsorship arrangement was reached between Balloon Fiesta organizers and Kimberly-Clark whereby a diaper-changing tent was placed on the spectator grounds; the tent featured comfortable changing tables, complimentary diapers, wipes, diaper rash ointment, and diaper pails. In exchange for their event association, the sponsor provided the Balloon Fiesta organization with an undisclosed amount of money (Turco, 1994).

Step 2. Secure media sponsors. Television, radio, and print media businesses should be approached before other prospective sponsors because they can serve a dual purpose for the sport event organization: (a) creating event awareness among spectator markets and (2) providing operating resources (e.g., money, volunteers).

Step 3. Define sponsorship levels. It is important to describe for the buyer (prospective corporate sponsor) the sponsorship opportunities and benefits available. After all, the corporation needs to know what it is buying. Examples of sponsorship opportunities may include title sponsorship, product category exclusivity, or "presenting" sponsor designations. For example, a variety of sponsorship levels are available for the Albuquerque International Balloon Fiesta. These different sponsorship levels have market values (in dollars) corresponding with the benefits to be received.

Step 4. Develop sponsorship proposal. Prospective sponsors may or may not be aware of an event that is "for sale." Therefore, it behooves the event marketer to provide prospective buyers with enough information so that they may make an informed purchase decision. A sponsorship proposal typically includes the following information:

- description of event organization;
- description of the event itself
- sponsor benefits/levels

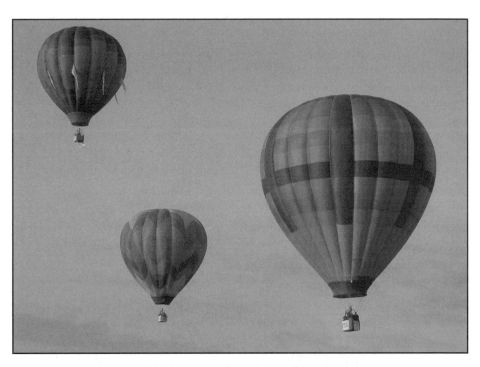

Sponsors must consider what kinds of benefits they want before they decide how much they want to spend.
Photo reprinted by permission of Jackie Kurkowski.

- media and promotional plans

- impact measurement

- appendices

Step 5. Identify and target prospective sponsors. The following questions may assist the event marketer in identifying prospective sport sponsors:

1. What products or services does the targeted company produce?

2. What are the characteristics of the target's consumers?

3. What are the general promotional approaches of the target company?

    a. Where does the company stand versus the competition?

    b. Has the company used sport or event sponsorship before?

        If yes, was the experience positive or negative?

        Has the company previously sponsored the event you are representing? Was the relationship positive?

    c. Who makes the marketing decisions for the target company?

4. Why would this company want to sponsor this event/service?

5. What possible controversies might result from this company's sponsorship of the event/service?

6. How will an event/service benefit from a sponsorship arrangement with this business?

Who Makes Sponsorship Decisions?

Weppler and McCarville (1994) attempted to better understand the corporate decision-making process with regard to involvement in fairs, festivals, and special events. Using a qualitative approach, this research focused on corporate decision-makers' beliefs, ideas, and biases in relation to sport sponsorship. In-depth interviews with event sponsors demonstrated that buying centers or committees were very typical in the evaluation of sponsorships. Four members were common to most buying centers. Those members and the specific roles they played are described in the following paragraph. It is important to note that the members of these groups varied with the complexity of the sponsorship.

For the roles played by individuals in buying centers, "Gatekeepers" were those individuals who made the decision on what and how much information was passed on to key decision-makers. These individuals were the committee members who received the initial sponsorship proposal. Gatekeepers included receptionists, assistants, and even consulting firms. "Influencers" were those individuals who had some sort of connection or information regarding the sponsorship requester. Most often the influencer was outside of the buying center. Included in this group of individuals were senior managers, other company employees, or friends who had experienced past events put on by the sponsorship requester. The ultimate decision-makers, or "deciders," varied depending on the level and cost of the sponsorship. Small sponsorship proposals were often referred to local or regional managers, whereas larger, more lucrative proposals were handled by the corporate staff. The final role was that of the buyer. The main responsibility of this position was to undertake negotiations with the event manager. Negotiations were undertaken to ensure that the corporations interests were being met (Weppler & McCarville, 1994).

McCook, Turco, and Riley (1997) found that large, national companies used a gatekeeper as the initial sponsorship decision-maker. These gatekeepers were most often advertising agency representatives, who decide whether or not to pass a sponsorship opportunity on to key decision-makers. The key decision-makers usually include the advertising department's senior management or department heads. The ultimate decision-

It is important for sport marketers who are seeking corporate sponsors to learn as much as possible about what companies look for when making sponsorship decisions. From initial meetings with a business's decision-makers and through secondary intelligence gathering, a thorough understanding of the company's objectives, prior to the development of the sponsorship proposal, is important to the success of the plan for a sport marketer. By gaining an understanding of each individual company and of its mission and markets, a sponsorship can be developed to meet specific corporate needs. Once a proposal is accepted, client service and/or followup are of utmost importance in making company decision-makers feel satisfied with their sponsorship decision and, it is hoped, in guaranteeing a renewal. Preferred client service/followup included occasional contact with the company representative to be sure the company is happy with the sponsorship. It is important to make sure the sponsorship is running smoothly in the eyes of the client. Without followup, a sport marketer may find out about sponsorship problems after it is too late to make amends. Offering clients game tickets, tournament tickets, and special event opportunities can help to make them feel as if they are a part of the sport "team." As with any sale, it is important to build good rapport with the client and make them feel comfortable with their sport sponsorship decision. A sound business relationship and personal rapport with sponsor clients can be simply attained through periodic contact and correspondence. High turnover at the regional levels of some corporations makes this difficult, as the sponsorship decision-maker may change on a seemingly annual basis. Sport marketers should place greater emphasis on sponsorship retention as it is five times more expensive to attract a new sponsor than to retain an existing sponsor (Turco, 1999).

makers depend on the level and cost of the sponsorship. Small sponsorships were often handled by local managers or an advertising director, whereas larger sponsorship opportunities were brought before the vice-president of the department and his or her committee. The decision-making process for small, local companies differed in that decisions were made by the store owner or manager. These people were responsible not only for making the sponsorship decision but also for operating the company. Once again, the decision-maker varied, depending on the size (in dollars) of the sponsorship opportunity. Decisions on small sponsorships are typically made by the local manager, whereas larger, more costly decisions require the inclusion of the owner of the company. These results closely matched those of the study conducted by Weppler and McCarville (1994) regarding the corporate decision-making process for events and festivals. Sport marketers should seek to identify the key decision-maker when proposing a sponsorship opportunity to a business, and not deal initially with clerks or assistant managers.

Sport Tour: NASCAR Is Moving Up

NASCAR, the acronym for the National Association Stock Car Automobile Racing, is on an economic roll, fueled by fan interest. More than 5.8 million fans attended the 32 Winston Cup races in 1995, up 66% since 1990; an additional 160 million watched on five broadcast and cable-television networks. During the same period, NBA attendance rose 17%, NFL was up 6%, and Major League Baseball was up 5.8%.

In 1997, Daytona International Speedway added another 18,000 seats and built 24 new hospitality suites. Richmond is building 12,000 new seats. Phoenix is adding another 25,000. Darlington is building a new 7,500-seat tower. Bristol Motor Speedway is expanding to 131,000 seats and adding 75 more luxury suites.

Sponsors are quickly learning that activating a NASCAR integrated sponsorship not only generates more sales but also allows for more creative ways to get their message across to consumers. One case in point is Anheuser-Busch.

In the early 1990s, sales of canned beer declined about 10%, compared with bottled beer. A-B wanted to reverse this trend, and targeted its Busch brand for a special campaign using NASCAR's integrated sponsorship program. The strategy was to use a popular driver and familiar racetracks to promote special commemorative cans. Dale Earnhardt starred in a series of TV commercials that profiled colorful tracks, including Darlington and Bristol. Since the introduction of the program, sales of Busch beer in cans have grown 7%, a 17-point swing from the competition. NASCAR is so confident of the value of its integrated approach that it plans to develop racing-related themes for combined marketing impact. Each year, the entire sport will be focused on one overall theme, in effort to provide sponsors with an integrated, coordinated platform for their promotions.

Sponsorship Considerations

Sponsorship deals, particularly those at five-figure dollar levels and above, are often based upon the rapport/relationship between buyer and seller. McCook et al. (1997) recommend that the sport marketer use previously established contacts to schedule meetings with targeted business decision-maker(s).

It is also recommended that the marketer submit a written sponsorship plan to the targeted corporate decision-maker in advance of an arranged meeting. During the meeting with the sponsorship decision-maker(s), the marketer should be flexible in the approach to the sponsorship sales. If the sponsor prospect is hesitant to commit to an initial agreement, the marketer should, if possible, offer alternative arrangements to meet corporate needs. It is further recommended that a followup letter be sent to the corporate decision-maker, restating the key points from the meeting. Once an agreement has been reached, a written sponsorship contract should be prepared with the following items specified:

- Benefits to the sponsoring business

- Terms of sponsorship

- Exclusivity

- Licenses and use of marks

- Payment schedules

- Dates for deliverables

- Breach of contract

- Renewals

- Sponsorship evaluation

Businesses prefer to see sponsorship costs, length of contract, value-added promotions, and media coverage in a sponsorship proposal (McCook, Turco & Riley, 1997). It is important for sport marketers to make an effort to work with businesses to create sponsorships that mutually benefit the cooperating organizations (Stotlar & Kadlecek, 1993). Multiyear "flex" deals allow organizers the advantage of long-term sponsorships and corporations the opportunity to adjust the nature and objectives of their promotion on an annual basis if desired.

Sport Sponsorship Issues

Several sport sponsorship issues with implications to sport tourism marketers are covered in this section. One issue relates to the compatibility or appropriateness of the sport and sponsor. We call this the sport-sponsor "fit." A good sport-sponsor fit might be a professional beach volleyball association tournament and a sunscreen producer. A poor sport-sponsor fit would involve a liquor store and a Little League baseball team. Poor public image and reduced product sales are consequences of poor sport-sponsor fit.

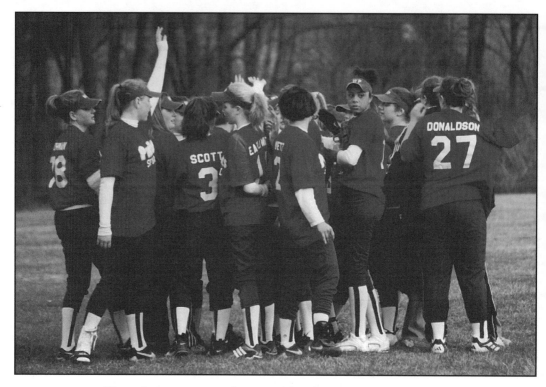

***Choosing an appropriate sponsor for a team is essential
to maintain a good public image.***

Photo reprinted by permission of Jackie Kurkowski.

The sport marketplace has become cluttered with sport sponsorship opportunities, and there is a growing anti-commercialism sentiment
among some spectators and event organizers. They see the number of
signs, logos, and sponsorship intrusions made upon the contest itself as
excessive and long for a purer game void of such distractions. A consumer backlash due to sport overcommercialization may ensue. Sponsorship clutter limits the effectiveness of sport as a promotional vehicle
for all sponsors. A fine line exists between satisfying the bottom line for
an event organization through sponsorship dollars and alienating fans
due to over-commercializing the event. When an event organization offers a sponsor benefits in exchange for resources, it relinquishes some
control to the sponsor.

One of the most publicized sport sponsorship issues involves the tobacco industry. In 1996, tobacco firms devoted 95% of their $195 mil-
lion sports sponsorship budget to motor sports (*IEG*, 1997). R.J.
Reynolds, producer of Winston cigarettes, is one of the most prominent

**Tobacco
Sponsorship
in Sport**

names in auto racing and spends approximately $30 million annually on motor sports advertising and promotion, including the Winston Cup and other NASCAR events. Other tobacco makers provide another 20% of sponsorship money for motor sports. Tobacco's forced exit may create opportunities for new sponsorship entries in sport. NASCAR's surging attendance, TV ratings and merchandise sales have attracted a wide range of sponsors, including McDonald's, Coca-Cola, and Kodak, corporations that could compensate if tobacco firms are driven from racetracks. The tobacco industry has developed a strong relationship with several sports organizations due, in part, to the 1971 ban on television and radio advertising, a result of the Public Health Smoking Act of 1970 (Madden & Grube, 1994).

Using sport sponsorship, tobacco messages have still found their way on television. Examining over 100 televised sporting events from 1990 to 1992, Madden and Grube (1994) found indirect tobacco messages and images appeared on television an average of 1.5 times per hour, in essence circumventing the purpose of the 1971 ban on television advertising.

In 1998, Texas, Florida, Minnesota, and Mississippi each won separate court settlements with the tobacco industry, receiving a total of $39.1 billion to recover money spent on treating sick smokers. The Texas settlement was worth $15 billion and required that all tobacco-related billboards in Texas be eliminated. However, the settlement did allow tobacco companies to keep their sponsorships, such as NASCAR's Winston Cup. Texas tried, but was unable, to have those sponsorships banned. The European Union, however, banned tobacco sponsorship in 1997, and Formula One racing has until 2006 to remove its tobacco advertising.

Free speech advocates have argued that under the First Amendment, the tobacco industry has the right to advertise its products on television or radio. Various levels of the U.S. judicial system have upheld decisions that commercial advertisers are not covered by the First Amendment (Turco, 1999). The tobacco industry argues that tobacco is a legal product, and therefore, the industry has every right to promote that product, as long as the promotions are not aimed at minors. Critics of tobacco sponsorship in sport point to the high percentage of spectators viewing events, in person or through other media services, who are under the age of 18 (Turco, 1999). These critics argue that the frequency of tobacco advertising in sports has triggered an increase in youth smoking rates.

It is clear that in the future, sport marketers will have to sever their ties with the tobacco industry. The ban on tobacco sponsorship in sport will allow other companies to capitalize on the opportunities to enter into, or invest more in, sponsorship. Turco (1999) surmises that other industries will fill the sponsorship void left by the tobacco industry, and the sporting world will hardly notice the difference.

Bonds

General funds are typically used to meet operating needs (e.g., salaries, equipment, supplies). Most major long-term expenditures incurred by the public sector (capital development projects) are paid for through the sale of bonds. Bonds are formally defined as a promise to pay back a specified amount of money, with interest, within a specified period of time. Essentially, a bond is an interest-paying IOU. The interest is expressed as a percentage of the principal (face amount of the bond) available for use during a specified period. Many high school athletic facilities that attract nonresident participants and spectators are financed through general obligation bonds after successful voter referenda.

Kraus (1997) describes the process of the sale of bonds as follows:

> Basically, this involves the agency obtaining legal authorization (generally from the voters and/or the local legislative authority) to borrow money from a qualified lender. The lender can be any individual, organization, or group with money to lend at interest. Usually this is an established financial institution such as a bank, an investment service, or sometimes an insurance company. When the financial institution lends the money to the public agency, the agency provides the lender with an appropriate number of engraved certificates (usually issued in $1,000 or $5,000 denominations). These redeemable certificates, or bonds, represent the legal obligation of the public agency (borrower) to pay back the bond holder (the lending institution) the amount borrowed, together with a fixed interest rate. (p. 11)

Types of bonds. There are basically two types of bonds issued by the public sector for sport facility development: general obligation bonds and revenue bonds. The basic difference between these bonds can be explained by the source of money used to pay them back. A general obligation bond is paid back through general property taxes. A revenue bond is a form of nonguaranteed debt that is retired from money generated by the facility that was built by bond money.

The sale of general obligation bonds usually requires voter approval because it leads to an increase in local taxes. Writes Kraus:

> In the case of a general obligation bond, the borrower (city, county, school district) pledges the full faith and credit of its taxing power to the bondholder. In effect, the governmental unit makes an unconditional promise to pay back the interest and principal owed, through its authority to levy taxes (p. 12).

The primary requirement for using revenue bonds is, obviously, that the proposed facility can generate enough money to meet operating costs and pay back the debt. Prior to issuing the revenue bonds, the government entities involved usually commission a feasibility to determine whether the community will use and pay for the facility. Another strategy used with revenue bonds is to back the bonds with income from another revenue stream, with lodging taxes being a popular source (Howard & Crompton, 1995).

Funding for Nonprofit Organizations

Numerous sport organizations in the United States operate under the classification of nonprofit status. Although most of the aforementioned revenue sources are used by nonprofit organizations (NPOs), their unique status affords them several financial benefits. NPOs are classified in the legal sense by both state law and federal Internal Revenue Service (IRS) code. Organizations are classified and categorized with varying benefits and restrictions in accordance with their mission, types of services, whether there is an intent to make a profit, and so on. In awarding an organization nonprofit status, the IRS lays out two benefits. First, it exempts certain classes of nonprofit organizations from taxation on the profits

A Comparison of General Obligation and Revenue Bonds

General Obligation Bonds	Revenue Bonds
Advantages	*Advantages*
1. Recreation is an essential government service deserving of tax support	1. Only the users pay for the bonds
2. Easier to sell because of comparatively reduced risk of default	2. No referendum for voter approval is required—facilitates quick action by the local administration
3. Lower interest rates than revenue bonds	3. Not included in statutory debt limitations
4. Allows services to be provided on the basis of need, not profit	*Disadvantages*
Disadvantages	1. Higher interest rates
1. Favorable election referendum necessary	2. Harder to sell because of uncertainty factors of
2. Increases the local tax burden	a. weather
3. Contribute to the legal debt of the issuing	b. competition
	c. voluntary participation
	3. Increases risk of default
	4. May restrict participation because of higher user fees

received in the business. Second, it establishes that donations or gifts to specified types of nonprofit organizations are deductible from the donor's taxable income. Nonprofit sport organizations, particularly those facilitating participatory sport tourism experiences, are eligible for most grants whereas for-profit organizations may be excluded from consideration. For example, the Illinois Department of Natural Resources and the Illinois Department of Transportation provide matching grants to municipal park and recreation departments to construct trail systems on abandoned railways for inline skating, bicycling, jogging, and exercise walking.

Each of the different classes of NPOs under the IRS code has benefits and stipulations that correspond to its particular section code. The many varying classes of NPOs are recognized by the IRS and described in Sections 501(a) through 501(h) of the tax code. Nonprofit organizations may be divided into two types, those under Section 501(c)(3) and those not under that classification of the tax code.

NPOs classified under Section 501(c)(3) are exempt from federal income taxation on certain forms of income received by the organization, and donors are entitled to tax deductions on donations and contributions. NPOs other than those in Section (c) (3) are granted exemption from income taxation under the code, but donations and contributions do not entitle donors to a tax deduction. To qualify for favored tax treatment, nonprofit organizations must be dedicated to furthering a public charitable purpose rather than private gain, have its mission fall within the specific classifications of exempt charitable purpose established by the IRS, and accept certain restrictions on its political activities (Kraus & Curtis, 2000).

Government funding is a very viable source of revenue for many NPOs, and, in some cases, is vital to the overall success of the agency. Corporate support via foundation grants is another major source of funding for nonprofit leisure services agencies. Many corporations provide financial support for charitable activities, as the federal tax code permits businesses to deduct a portion of their gross income for gifts to charities.

Sport tourism organizations seeking corporate foundation resources should be aware of several considerations. Corporations tend to favor supporting organizations in close geographic proximity to their headquarters or branch offices. Corporations favor a sport service that is directly needed or consumed by their organization (e.g., child care for working couples or single-parent employees). Third, it is also helpful to have "connections" with persons of authority in a corporation who may advocate the sport tourism proposal.

Family foundations, community foundations, and individual donations are other sources of funding for the nonprofit leisure services organizations. Family foundations number over 20,000 and are commonly created in memory of a deceased family member. Individual donations represent between 50 and 85% of the total funding for nonprofit agencies. An important part of raising funds from individuals is the tax benefits donors receive from their charitable contribution.

Grants

Grants for sport tourism operations are more likely for NPOs than for for-profit organizations. The application process for foundation grant support is similar to that for public sector grants. There are six interrelated steps to successful grant writing (Smith & McLean, 1988):

1. Idea formulation

2. Selection of external funding source

3. Proposal preparation

4. Proposal submission

5. Proposal acceptance or rejection

6. Grant administration or proposal revision and resubmission.

As the grant experience is started, several questions need to be answered before actually beginning the grant proposal. Answering these questions at the very beginning of the process will save much time, effort, and frustration later on.

Question 1. Are the chances of your proposal being funded good enough to be worth your time and effort?

Question 2. Is your grant proposal in harmony with your personal and professional goals, and does it meet the philosophy and goals of your agency?

Question 3. Can this project be accomplished without hindering the goals, direction, and function of the agency?

Question 4. Why are you undertaking this adventure? Are you being honest and realistic with yourself and your agency?

Several online databases can assist the sport tourism manager in identifying granting organizations including the Foundation Center (www.fdncenter.org), Foundations Online (www.foundations.org/page2.html), Grants Web (web.fie.com/cws/sra/resource.htm), and the Grantsmanship Center (www.tgci.com). In the past, foundations for Hershey Chocolate, American Express, and State Farm Insurance have provided financial resources for sport operations.

Among revenue-generating strategies, property tax levies continue to be the method of choice for local governments in raising revenue for sport tourism operations. Other government taxes to finance sport tourism operations include alcohol, tobacco, and sport/recreation equipment sales taxes. Park district, hotel/motel, and recreation district taxes are also among the most prevalent types of special taxation utilized to finance sport operations.

There are seven classifications of fees and charges in sport administration: (a) entrance fees, (b) admission fees, (c) rental fees, (d) user fees, (e) sales revenues, (f) license and permit fees, and (7) special service fees. There are six general pricing methods used in determining fees for the delivery of sport services: (a) marginal cost pricing, (b) full pricing, (c) differential pricing, (d) traditional pricing, (e) going-rate pricing, and (f) equity pricing.

Many sport tourism development projects are paid for through the sale of bonds. Bonds may be defined as a promise to pay back a specified amount of money, with interest, within a specified period of time. There are two major types of bonds issued by the public sector: *general obligation bonds and revenue bonds*. A general obligation bond is paid back through general property taxes; a revenue bond is retired from money generated by the facility that is built by the bond money.

Summary

International Events Group, Inc. (IEG)

Sponsorship Resources

640 North LaSalle, Suite 600
Chicago, IL 60610-3777 U.S.A.
Telephone: 1.800.834.4850 (outside the United States, call 312.944.1727)
Fax: 312.458.7111; E-mail: ieg@sponsorship.com
www.sponsorship.com

International Festivals and Events Association (IFEA)

P.O. Box 2950
115 E. Railroad Ave., Suite 302
Port Angeles, WA 98362
TEL: 360.457.3141 FAX: 360.452.4695
www.ifea.com

Chapter 8

Professional Preparation in Sport Tourism

Questions

1. What are the basic academic competencies in sport and tourism necessary for professional preparation in sport tourism?
2. What are the benefits to students involved with a service learning experience in sport tourism?
3. What are the benefits of active membership in sport tourism professional associations?

Introduction

The most obvious time for preparation to face the professional world is after high school and college. There is also a need for professional preparation or retooling during employment transitions. School-ending transitions are the result of a natural progression, but the other transitions occur after becoming disappointed with a career choice, being "let go" from an existing position, or when seeking professional growth and challenge. Before heading for positions in the sports tourism field, it would be a good investment to research the employment situation thoroughly to find out about job availability.

According to Farr, Ludden, and Mangin (1997), there are several considerations when people find themselves in the transition of job seeking. Sport tourism services providers are known for their long work hours. First, the job seeker must investigate the nature of the work he or she will be doing. Job seekers must know the duties to be performed, the complexity and variety of tasks, the hours of labor, the level of responsibility and accountability, and the intensity of supervision. Given a thorough understanding of these variables, job seekers will be able to assess the level of knowledge they need to acquire, the skills they need to demonstrate, and the abilities required for success in their chosen sports tourism position. Second, prospective job seekers should research the employment outlook before gaining the necessary knowledge, skills, and abilities. There would be nothing worse than investing in several years of education to improve one's knowledge, only to find that few positions exist in one's chosen field. For instance, positions with professional or collegiate sports teams are rare and difficult to obtain. Finally, job seekers must assess the earnings potential of any position to see whether it will meet their fiscal needs. When doing so, one must be sure to account for low-level salaries at the entry level. One must also account for salary potential after advancing to higher ranks. For some people, salaries are not as important as job satisfaction whereas for others, salary is crucially important so they can maintain a healthy lifestyle.

This chapter on professional development presupposes an interest in sport tourism. No matter the academic environment, good grades are only part of what it takes to enter the sports tourism profession. This statement is meant not to diminish the value of an education, but to alert people to other necessities that must be fulfilled. Because this field of study and work is highly competitive and applied, there is a strong need for people to look beyond university courses to practicums, internships, summer jobs, and volunteerism to complete their professional preparation. During these practical episodes of education, people not only can apply what they have learned in the class but also can make contacts with the industry. It should also be noted that professional development does not stop once the first position is obtained. Professionals need to keep abreast of trends in the field and must keep professionally connected.

This chapter, therefore, looks at professional development in with two items in mind. It will look at the variety of educational choices when pursuing a career in sports tourism, and it will look at various strategies for staying current and keeping professionally connected with the field.

Academic Programs

Academic programs specifically designed for sport tourism are hard to find, but their development is inevitable given the growth of the industry. At the present time, students who wish to study sports tourism must house themselves in one of a variety of programs that teach courses related to both tourism and sports. Students of sport tourism will most often find themselves in sports management programs, tourism programs, recreation and leisure studies programs, or business programs that concentrate on sports or tourism, or both. The ideal situation at this time would be a double major in sports management and tourism although a major in one with a minor in the other would also suffice. The next most preferable situation would be a major in a business or leisure/recreation program where an emphasis or specialization in sports management or tourism can be obtained.

In all the options listed above, the World Wide Web is the student's greatest ally. Many academic Web sites are devoted to listing programs that may suit their academic needs. If the student is already in a program, these sites may be useful when choosing a master's or doctoral program. Listed below is a comprehensive but incomplete set of Web resources that can guide students to sports management, tourism, and recreation/leisure studies programs. According to Parkhouse (1996), there were over 200 sport management degree programs in the United States alone whereas there are an equal number of tourism programs.

Websites for Sports Management/ Tourism/ Recreation Programs: Undergraduate and Graduate

www.unb.ca/SportManagement/programs.htm.
The University of Northern British Columbia (Canada) site provides for links to sport management programs in Australia, Canada, Europe, and the United States. The table listing the programs also indicates whether the programs offer undergraduate, graduate or doctoral degrees.

ace.acadiau.ca/spmg/portfol.htm
This Acadia University (Canada) site provides links to graduate programs in sport management.

playlab.uconn.edu/phdprogs.htm
The University of Connecticut (US) site provides links to doctoral programs in sport management, tourism, leisure studies, and the sociology of sport.

www.geog.ualbeta.ca.als/rlsres.html
This is entitled "Recreation and Leisure Studies: Resources on the World Wide Web." The site is housed at the University of Alberta (Canada). It offers a listing of academic programs in recreation, leisure, and tourism. Many of these programs also offer sport management degrees. The programs are listed by countries that include Australia, Austria, Canada, Netherlands, New Zealand, United Kingdom, and United States.

www.msu/edu/~dopplick/
The "Official Tourism Sources Worldwide" offers links to recreation/ leisure studies sites in the United States and tourism programs worldwide. Web surfers need to click on "Academia" to retrieve these sites. Beware: The "academia" icon is very hard to see on the main page. Listings of tourism programs include the countries of Australia, Austria, Canada, Egypt, England, Germany, Netherlands, New Zealand, and Scotland.

sfbox.vt.edu:10021/Y/yfleung/recres2.html

Located at the University of Vermont, the "Natural Resources: Research Information Pages" list academic and educational sites worldwide in the fields mentioned above.

Countries include Australia, Austria, Canada, Netherlands, New Zealand, South Africa, Taiwan, Thailand, United Kingdom, and United States.

www.lin.ca

Located in Canada, the Leisure Information Network lists many academic programs in several countries.

Although all these sites list many academic programs in sports management, tourism, and recreation/leisure studies, people seeking a particular type of program will have to research the programs to find the best match. The newest offering that deals with sport tourism degrees directly is the program being developed by the CSM—Institute of Graduate Studies in cooperation with the Sports Tourism International Council (STIC) located in Canada. Degrees in sport tourism will be offered at the associate, baccalaureate, master's and doctoral levels, with specializations in sports events, sports tours, sports attractions, sports resorts and sports cruises. Various experts in the field will offer these degrees through distance learning technologies. To find out more about the development of these programs, students should visit <www.sportsquest.com/tourism/index.html>.

Those who already have experience in the area of sport tourism may be more attracted by the forthcoming certification program that will be offered by the same organizations. This Web site also discusses the certification initiatives.

Core Content of Undergraduate Studies

Because sport tourism as an area of study is so new, students are best to combine courses in sport management and tourism programs to give themselves the overview they need. There are but a few sport tourism specialists degree programs offered worldwide, including the University of Luton (United Kingdom) and Southern Cross University (Australia). Core content areas at the undergraduate level have been described in the United States by a joint taskforce. The contributing bodies of this taskforce were the North American Society for Sport Management (NASSM) and the National Association for Sport and Physical Education (NASPE). From this joint venture, 10 content areas were deemed important for sport management students.

1. Behavioral dimensions in sport

2. Management and organizational skills in sport

3. Ethics in sport management

4. Marketing in sport

5. Communication in sport

6. Finance in sport

7. Economics in sport

8. Legal aspects in sport

9. Governance in sport

10. Field experience in sport (Parkhouse, 1996).

The content areas do not specify particular courses but areas that need to be covered. Some departments of sport management cover all these content areas themselves, and other use different departments to cover some of the specialist areas.

Although the various academic programs offering sport management deal with this outline in different ways, the outline does little to address tourism needs. At this stage there are no nationally or internationally recognized content guidelines set forth on core content areas. However, some individuals have attempted to outline the various academic aspects that are needed. Perhaps Hudman and Hawkins (1989) offer the most easily understandable model of the knowledge. Their model has four major components with various subsections in each component. The four major components and associated sub sections are depicted in Table 8.1.

Somewhere between these suggested content areas is a plan of study that would suit the sport tourism student. By comparing the NASPE model to the one by Hudman and Hawkins (1989), it can be seen that the areas of human behaviors and motivations, and all the elements of the business environment are commonalties within both outlines. However, even in these areas of similarity, there are many differences in practice and process that are situation specific. Where these programs of study do find very similar requirements is in their service learning modules. The following section outlines the benefits of service learning and offers some Web sites to search for internship possibilities.

Table 8.1. Content Areas of Academic Programs in Tourism

Component 1: Dynamic Element—The Tourism Phenomenon
Basic Concepts, Principles and History of Tourism—Factors Influencing Travel in General

Component 2: Services Element—The Tourism System

Tourism Demand
— tourist motivation and behavior

Linkages between Supply and Demand
— communications and promotion
— transportation and tour operations
— distribution channels and pricing strategies

Tourism Supply
— attractions
— lodging and food services
— visitor services
— meeting and facility services
— public and private tourism organizations

Component 3: Functional Element—Tourism Management

Research and Forecasting for Tourism

Tourism Policy and Regulation

Tourism Planning

Tourism Marketing

Education and Training for Tourism

Component 4: Consequential Element—Tourism Impacts

Economic Impacts

Social and Cultural Impacts

Environmental Impacts

Service Learning: Internships, Practicums, and Fieldwork Experiences

As with most applied degrees, time working with professionals is invaluable for putting theory into practice. Without practice, theory has little context and therefore may be understood incompletely. These theoretical or conceptual understandings may also be given different levels of importance when compared with what happens in the "real world." The practical nature of service learning acts as a modifying and balancing force to situate the theoretical and conceptual components. Furthermore, when learning the concepts and theories of sport tourism, students are likely to be imbued with the best case scenarios, or how things would work in a perfect world if there were no constraints or resource shortages. Through service learning, students will understand that there is no perfect world, that plenty of constraints and resource shortages are common. They will be able to see how the professional deals with these challenges and changes on a daily basis.

From a more bloody-minded viewpoint, there is little use obtaining a degree in sport, tourism, or sport tourism if students have not gotten their "hands dirty." Indeed, there is little use in the degree without a practical experience because few employers will want to hire students without experience. It is here that fieldwork, internships, and practica play their part. These service learning experiences have other benefits also. They provide the student with portfolio-building experiences and add to their professional network base when searching for that first position.

The benefits of service learning experiences, according to Verner (1996), apply to three constituents even though the students are the focus. Receiving benefits from these experiences are students, the sponsoring educational programs, and the organization that hosts students.

Students accrue the benefits of service learning opportunities from several places:

- New learning environments—People learn their knowledge and skills in different ways, and internships provide another way to learn. This learning opportunity occurs outside the safe environment of the classroom but allows the use of classroom knowledge to be put into practice. The most important part of the "real world" environment is that students' actions (work) will have real implications and consequences. They are confronted with the need to problem solve and make several decisions that affect other people. This responsibility directly contrasts the educational environment in which students are accountable only to themselves.

- Professional commitment and accountability—A glamorized view of the sport tourism profession is easy to gain in classroom settings. When choosing to research and write papers, students will most often choose exciting rather than mundane subjects. When completing an internship, however, students are subjected to the routine, the unpleasant, and the boring aspects of their profession. These service learning opportunities give students a full view of their field. With commitments to other people, the intern also discovers they are accountable for their actions and not just their grade. Sometimes this accountability factor will demand the need for odd hours, long hours, and unpleasant work. At the end of it all, students can make decisions about their continued interest in sport tourism, or in the particular area of sport tourism they find most interesting.

- Self-Assessment in the "battlefield"—Although the internship is a training ground, it is also a testing ground. Not only can students assess their knowledge, skills, and abilities, but supervising professionals will also evaluate them. With self-assessments and external assessments, students become armed with information about their strengths and weaknesses that will allow them to highlight the former and improve the latter.

- Portfolio enhancement—The harsh reality of the work world is that, to get a job one needs experience, and to get experience one needs . . . there seems little point to finishing this "Catch 22" situation. The wonderful aspect of internships is their provision of job experience that can be documented and presented to potential employers. In applied professions such as sport tourism, work experience is important, and the internship opportunity should be a capstone experience along with lesser experiences of practica, fieldwork, volunteerism, and summer employment. A portfolio with a variety of work experiences will serve students well.

- Evaluation of career settings—Although late in the academic experience, internships allow students to evaluate their career settings and choices. Based on their work-related experiences, they can position themselves where they best fit. On the other hand, they can receive feedback from agency supervisors about their strengths and weaknesses in particular sport tourism settings.

- Mentoring—Perhaps the greatest benefits of working with agency supervisors will come from their mentoring. Through these people, interns can learn their positions, receive advice on career trajectories, and gather strategies for development and professional improvement. Each professional can pass on mistakes and successes to the benefit of the interns.

- Networking—Internships provide immediate access to supervisors who can introduce interns to other professionals. These contacts can provide advice on career development, but more important, they may be prospective employers or people who can provide resources to get the job done. In a later section of this chapter, the art of networking will be discussed in greater depth.

- Unteachable situations—What professors and textbooks cannot teach are specific job duties, daily routines, crisis management, and the political permutations of every job. Each of these elements is situation specific and can be dealt with only through on-the-job experience. Although professors can provide knowledge, experience is the best teacher in these situations.

- Career launching—An internship is a stepping-stone to one's career. Internships provide practical experience, skill improvement, and networks with which to obtain the first position. From a successful internship comes an all-important letter of reference that may be the deciding factor for prospective employee.

For the sponsoring educational programs, service learning benefits can be accrued from

- Professional contact—Professors need contact with the "real world," too. Their positions at universities and colleges depend on the industries for which they train students. They must stay in contact to understand where the industry is heading and the situations it faces. Internships allow these contacts to be maintained through discussions with supervisors, reports from students, and on-site visits.

- Understanding current practices—In applied fields such as sport tourism, the envelope is pushed by the professionals more than academics. That is, everyday professionals are confronted with problems to which they must find solutions. By recognizing that professionals are innovators, professors can pass professional practices on to students. It behooves every professor to research internship sites for current practices, problems, and solutions so they can better serve their students.

- Course content enhancement—After researching the practices, problems, and solutions of the sport tourism field, professors can incorporate this knowledge into their classes to make learning more current and meaningful. They can achieve this by lecturing and by using examples, case studies, guest speakers, and assignments based on current practices.

- Enhanced "town and gown" relations—Through internships, university and college professors will create an impression with professionals. If favorable, the impression can enhance the job prospects of their students. If favorable, the professionals will be predisposed to take more interns and cooperate in other ways with the academic program.

- Potential research resources—The work world is the laboratory for professors in applied professions. Through internship contacts, professors can discover researchable problems and may receive funding to solve the research needs of professionals.

For the hosting organizations, service learning benefits can be accrued from

- Additional human resources—Internships are an exchange relationship from which students, university programs, and sponsoring agencies should benefit. One of the benefits returned to the agencies is the addition of human resources. Although resource-strapped agencies need interns to fulfill their professional obligations, it is preferable to think that most organizations request interns to enhance and expand the services they offer. Although both scenarios are true, neither scenario is true until the organization has trained an intern sufficiently.

- New ideas and skills—Often times interns have skills that are not available in the current staff. This is particularly true in today's technological age. Interns may be more computer literate than their professional colleagues and can therefore set up, maintain, and train full-time workers to exploit these technologies. When not encumbered by tradition and routine, students may view procedures and processes in a different way, questioning current practices and offering new solutions. Finally, agencies may benefit from the knowledge gained by students during their coursework. Although professionals are the innovators, college professors have compiled industry-wide knowledge for their students.

- Potential employment pools—By accepting interns, agencies have a steady string of potential employees they can evaluate without being obliged to employ. When the need arises, agencies have a chance to offer a position. The new employee's training has already occurred and he or she is immediately productive.

Finding internships is an area of expertise developed by most professors. However, students can widen this pool of choices by doing their own research. Once again, Web-based sites are the best technology for searching an array of choices. Listed below are sites specific to sport and tourism and sites that cover all types of internships. Also listed are the addresses of job bulletins that carry internship offerings.

Websites for Internships and Jobs

www.vicon.net/~internnet

When fully developed, Intern-NET will link students with internships all over the world. Its listings already include internships for students in sports, tourism, recreation and parks, hospitality and health-related professions. The site allows students to search by the aforementioned categories and by geographical preferences.

www.hrrm.psu.edu/JOBS.HTM

The Pennsylvania State University site links students to job listing and internship search mechanisms.

www.mysticseaport.org/williams-mystic/internships.html

The Maritime Studies Program of Williams College and Mystic Seaport has a number of internship sites and search engines for seeking out a service learning experience in sport tourism.

www.coolworks,com/showme

Coolworks is a site that has categories for seasonal positions in ski areas, national parks, cruises, and camps.

www.sponsorship.com/jobBank/jobBank.html

The IEG Job Bank has a place where prospective employees can submit their resumes, and there is a list of executive positions available in event and sports marketing.

www.ncaa.org/news/

For people interested in collegiate and university positions, most jobs are listed in the NCAA newsletter. Seek out the job listing in this publication.

www.onlinesports.com/pages/Resumes.html

The Online Sports Career Center has a place to deposit resumes so that prospective job seekers can view them.

www.sportslink.com/employment/jobs/index.html

This is the career center for the Sporting Goods Manufacturers Association.

wysiwyg://235/http://collegegrad.com/internships

The College.Grad.Job.Hunter site has a special page for students to search potential internships. Web surfers can browse the sites by key words.

National Sports Employment News

421 N. Northwest Highway, Suite 201, Barrington, IL 60010

National Recreation and Park Association—Job Bulletin

22377 Belmont Ridge Road, Ashburn, VA 20148-5401

Going to Graduate School

Some people may have a different degree before deciding on sport tourism as a profession, and other people may want to further their education in this field. However, going to graduate school is a very important decision. Individuals must have a clear idea of what they want to do before heading on for a master's or a doctoral degree. If the student is going directly to a master's degree from an undergraduate degree program, he or she must weigh the costs and benefits. On the one hand, these people will still be in the academic mode, but they will be short on work experience and will have to start at the bottom of the career ladder. On the other hand, they will have their advanced degrees already and will not have to go back for schooling later in life.

There are considerable benefits and costs when completing graduate degrees later in life. These people already have work experience, and they have professional networks to help them when they graduate. They will also be sure about the type of degree that will help them professionally upon graduation. It is highly likely that two degrees in sport tourism/sport management/tourism will not be beneficial. There are several costs to returning for an advanced degree after working for several years. Having become accustomed to a salary, many find it difficult to cut back on expenses to be a full-time student. There may also be financial and personal commitments that are difficult for a graduate student. The pluses and minuses must be worked through by each individual depending on personal circumstances and goals. Whatever the reasons are, it is not wise to complete another degree because one wishes to postpone working or because one is not sure about what one wants to do. Both reasons are recipes for disaster!

At this stage in the sport tourism field, there are only two reasons to pursue a doctoral degree. The first is to work as a professor of sport tourism at the college or university level. The second is to work as a researcher for a sport tourism company.

As opposed to undergraduate programs where the course content and the reputation of the school are important, at the advanced level, students should focus on their individual interests. These interests should be matched with the course offerings, but more important, people should match themselves with professors who have similar interests and expertise. Someone searching for a master's degree may find two types of graduate schools. The first is the master's program that aims students for placement in the profession and teaches the skills and knowledge to do so. The second are programs that focus on research. Once again, it becomes a matter of matching personal goals with the orientation and interests of the program and the professors. For a listing of graduate schools in sport management or tourism, use the same Web addresses provided earlier in this chapter.

When compared to those of undergraduate programs, admissions standards differ for master's or doctoral programs. First, master's and doctoral programs will have different requirements in terms of academic ability. Second, different universities will have different entrance requirements depending on their policies. The first step is to obtain all the requirements and standards so they are known. The second step is to assess whether these requirements can be met. The following research results may help prospective graduate students understand these requirements.

The requirements and standards for leisure studies doctoral programs were revealed in Arnold's (1994) study. Some of these programs had sport management degrees, and others had tourism degrees at both the master's and doctoral level. Although these results do not fit the exact mold of sport tourism, they indicate minimum requirements and expectations for entrance.

Arnold's (1995) study investigated four areas of admissions requirements: (a) academic preparation and achievement, (b) letters of recommendation, (c) standardized test scores, and (d) other favorable achievements (publications, presentations, and teaching experience). Eighty-seven percent of the schools considered the undergraduate grade point averages to be "moderately to extremely important," whereas all the schools cited master's degree grade point averages "moderately to extremely important." The academic reputation of undergraduate schools was less important whereas 75% cited the perceived quality of the graduate institution as "very important."

Letters of recommendation were another measure of a student's ability to perform academically. Letters of recommendation needed to be written by faculty members because letters from nonfaculty members held much less weight. Even more important, letters from faculty members known to the graduate program were more important than were letters from faculty who were not known.

The most influential measures of admission to programs were standardized test scores. All but one of the programs required Graduate Record Examination (GRE) scores, but other standardized tests (GMAT, MCAT) could be substituted. For foreign students, good TOEFL scores (550 and higher) were very important. The verbal and quantitative scores of the GRE were indicated to be most important whereas analytical scores were least important or not used by most institutions. Although the recommended minimum GRE scores averaged 530 for the verbal section and 500 for the quantitative, these scores fluctuated. Changes occurred when trying to control the size of enrollment and when candidates were being considered for graduate assistantships and scholarships. Graduate schools, especially for Ph.D.-granting programs, also stated that prior publications, professional presentations, and to a lesser extent, previous teaching experience were extremely influential in the decision-making process. A profile of an average successful graduate applicant had criteria such as

1. At least a 3.0 undergraduate GPA and 3.4 graduate GPA (on a 4-point scale)

2. 1030 combined on the verbal and quantitative sections of the GRE examination.

Arnold (1995) cited two additional concerns when applying for graduate school. These two factors were grade inflation and gender bias. Because grade inflation is an issue in college and universities, undergraduate and master's degree GPAs are less important than they once were. With inflated GPAs there is little differentiation between high-performing and low-performing undergraduates. This problem has created a reliance on standardized scores even though it has been argued that they are not good indicators of future performance. The reliance on test scores leads to the other issue. According to Sadker and Sadker (1994), females score lower than males do on the GRE by 127 points. It is difficult to verify this information because 1987–1988 was the last year the Educational Testing Service revealed information pertaining to these scores.

When the education is complete, it is time to seek a job in the field. This transition requires preparation and persistence because many competitors are doing exactly the same thing. To stand out from the crowd, job seekers should be thorough in their search.

Seeking Employment

When seeking a job in sport tourism, candidates may have to settle for the job they can obtain to receive the job that they want. In other words, people need to "get their foot in the door," perform well, develop good networks, and gain experience before they can compete for the most appealing positions. Before doing any of these tasks, it is important to take a step back and conduct a personal inventory. The second step is to identify the organizations that meet personal and professional needs and seek out positions in these organizations. Most important, the third step is to prepare for life as a professional (Arnold & Bartlett, 1996; Seagle, Smith, & Dalton, 1992; Starr, 1993; Verner, 1996). Other important steps include writing good letters of inquiry and resumes, and developing strong interviewing skills, but there are several book references that can be used for these tasks.

When conducting personal inventories, job seekers must appraise their values, goals, skills, and strengths and weaknesses. Values relate to the things that are personally and professionally important. Here are some questions to ask:

1. Would I like to work for another or do I need to be my own boss?

2. Is money important or are there other professional importances that come before money?

3. Do I want to work in the public view or behind the scenes?

4. Do I want a routinized job or one with variety?

5. Is it important to stay in a particular geographical area, or am I willing to relocate?

Goals relate to preferred futures. They are professional achievements for the medium or long term. It is also important to set personal goals because they will affect professional aspirations and add balance to life in general. To ascertain professional goals, try answering these questions:

1. Do I want to be a frontline employee or a boss?

2. Do I want to work for other people or set up my own business?

3. How much money do I want to make?

4. Do I want to be a decision and vision maker, or do I want to follow other people?

Skills and knowledge acquisition are important to perform successfully. Most academic institutions provide job seekers with basic skills and knowledge, but they do not pretend to teach everything. Colleges and universities realize that each company does things differently and with a knowledge and skills base, employees should be able to learn these differences. Any assessment of knowledge and skills should return to the content outlines about sport management and tourism at the start of this chapter.

Assessments of strengths and limitations should be performed in relation to professional goals. Most people can readily identify their strengths but shy away from their limitations. It is good to realize limitations because they can be addressed in the future. With goals in mind, these questions may assist in assessing knowledge, skills and abilities:

1. Do I have the knowledge base to get the job I am seeking? Where do I feel very confident and where do I feel less confident?

2. Can I perform all the skills necessary to do the job successfully? Where do I feel very confident and where do I feel less confident?

3. Do I have the ability to do the job successfully? Where do I feel very confident and where do I feel less confident?

For entry-level people, answers might be difficult to ascertain without full-time work experience, but entry-level positions require less knowledge and fewer skills than do positions of experience. If candidates have undertaken several work and service learning experiences during their formal education, they will be less anxious about how they are going to achieve their goals.

The next step is to identify organizations that employ people in the types of positions sought. This is an important step because searching and communication will take time. It is hoped that some of this search can be undertaken as a part of an internship search. Luckily, the Internet allows job seekers to search a much wider array of organizations than were once available. There are many job sites on the Internet, but the best way to find a job is through your own network system. The U.S. Department of Labor (Starr, 1993) conducted research on how people find jobs, and the findings clearly show the benefits of networking:

- Of the job seekers studied, 34% found jobs through associates, friends, and relatives (personal and professional networks).

- Another 30% found jobs directly through employers (networks and service learning opportunities).

- 17% found jobs through advertisements (searching job listing).

- 7% found jobs through union hiring and other organizational connections.

- 6% found jobs through employment agencies.

- Another 6% found jobs through public employment agencies

With travel and tourism encompassing such a wide variety of employment opportunities, it can be difficult to determine which direction to head. Provided below are lists of employment locations to research when looking for a job. Before searching, the task is to list as many professional options as possible under each category and subcategory. This will indicate how well the job seeker knows the field of sport tourism.

Organizations Involved in Sport Tourism

Attractions

Natural Resource Areas

1. _____

2. _____

3. _____

Indoor Sports Areas

1. _____

2. _____

3. _____

Staged Sports Attractions

1. _____

2. _____

3. _____

Sports Commemoration Attractions

1. _____

2. _____

3. _____

Sports Hospitality Attractions

1. _____

2. _____

3. _____

Sports Resorts

1. _____

2. _____

3. _____

Organizations

Sports Associations

1. _____

2. _____

3. _____

Professional & Amateur League Offices

1. _____

2. _____

3. _____

Sports Organizing Committees

1. _____

2. _____

3. _____

Governmental Sports Promotion Bodies

1. _____

2. _____

3. _____

Travel Suppliers

Airlines

1. _____

2. _____

3. _____

Bus Tour Operators

1. _____

2. _____

3. _____

Cruises

1. _____

2. _____

3. _____

Sports Specialty Operators

1. _____

2. _____

3. _____

Upon obtaining a job or even when studying for a degree, one will find that the benefits of association membership are many. People in similar career fields form associations so they can collectively enhance their profession. Members of associations can receive a lot from joining, but they can give a lot to the profession by contributing to the association in some way. Associations may be local in their orientation but are often regional, national and international in their membership and links with other associations. Here are just a few of the benefits that can be received from association membership:

Professional Associations

1. Technical assistance—When you have a professional problem, a network of people within the association may have expertise in the problem area.

2. Publications—Magazines and newsletters keep professionals up-to-date with the latest challenges and trends.

3. Legislative lobbying—Associations keep abreast of any legislation that will negatively affect the profession or the people it serves. They will lobby governmental sources and provide legal assistance to fight any negative effects.

4. Conferences and business expos—Conferences help professionals to share their skills and knowledge with others and to view the latest products that assist with the work of the profession.

5. Meetings and seminars—Typically smaller than conferences, these gatherings provide specialty training and discussion in professional matters.

6. Funding sources and awards—Associations recognize their outstanding professionals with awards for excellence. They may also have foundations that provide scholarships for students or professional development funds for practitioners.

7. Certification—Associations will provide opportunities to become professionally certified and to maintain that professional certification through educational meetings. To have certification is a significant professional advantage when searching for new position and provides a credible professional standard.

8. Educational impact—Associations may require educational institutions to teach subject matter that is deemed necessary for incoming professionals, thereby protecting the profession and students in academic programs.

9. Discount buying and privileges—Because of membership numbers, many associations can broker purchasing arrangements far less expensive than those that can be bought individually.

10. Networking—The greatest benefit is that professional associations provide ready access to networking opportunities. These opportunities can lead to many types of professional development.

Because of the importance of networking, the next section is devoted to the art of networking. By engaging in these opportunities, an individual can find answers to problems, find jobs at the next level, and find opportunities to serve the field.

Networking

According to Arnold (1996), 8 out of 10 professionals advance their career by networking. Whether they are searching for a job, seeking to build community support, or widening professional contacts, the importance of networking is immeasurable. Attending state, regional, or national conferences provides an excellent opportunity for networking with other people in the profession because there is no better place to establish an array of contacts in one place.

Networking is best described as a process for developing and using contacts for information, advice, and support when pursuing professional challenges and opportunities. This process requires certain skills and techniques to be effective because networking is an *exchange* process. In order to get something from the contact, something must be given in return. The paybacks are rarely immediate as they occur over a long period of time. Therefore, network contacts must be maintained periodically. The following section offers some advice on developing and maintaining professional networks. This process should be started at the college or university level and continued for the rest of one's professional career.

Preconference Network Planning

Attending a conference is one of the few opportunities to make several contacts in a short period of time. To make the most of this time, be sure to get a conference agenda before the conference begins. Circle or highlight those sessions you want to attend or speakers you want to meet. At the on-site registration table, some conferences will provide lists of all the registrants along with their place of work. Highlight or circle the people you wish to meet during the conference. Some potential network contacts might include

• Educators at colleges and universities where you may do graduate work in the future. They can give you insight on how to be successful when applying to their program and provide information about the requirements and orientation of the program.

- Professionals who hold positions to which you aspire so that you can increase your knowledge about how to get there and later receive some mentoring from them. You may also be able to use this person as a resource for your own work or have him or her as a personal contact when you apply for a position within their organization.

- Professionals who hold job positions similar to your own so you can share ideas, strategies, and long-term goals for mutual benefit.

- Potential clients or consumers so you can assess their needs and wants before doing business with them.

- Politically connected people who hold powerful positions in your profession. These people can provide insight into current and future situations and may also be personal and professional allies in the future.

- People whose perspectives differ from your own to help you grow personally and professionally. By understanding differing viewpoints you gather a wider knowledge of issues and challenges that will make you more astute as a professional.

Evaluating Your Current and Future Network

This exercise will demonstrate to you the areas of strengths and weaknesses of your present network and may provide guidance for future networking goals. If their names are not known, indicate the positions or titles these people may hold.

Identify six people who have helped or will help you advance in your career. Describe how they have helped you, and describe how you can help them in return, now or in the future.

1. _____   2. _____   3. _____

4. _____   5. _____   6. _____

Identify three people in sports/tourism whom you respect and value as professionals. Describe the qualities that you admire.

1. _____   2. _____   3. _____

Identify three people in related fields who can help you get your job done. Describe how they can help you and how you can help them in return.

1. _____ 2. _____ 3. _____

Identify three people who can guide your career and provide you with professional mentoring and opportunities.

1. _____ 2. _____ 3. _____

Identify three people who advise you of opportunities and encourage your professional visibility. How can you enhance their visibility?

1. _____ 2. _____ 3. _____

With the network targets identified, it is time to make and maintain some professional contacts. Despite the superficiality of first impressions, they clearly moderate how you will be regarded in the future. Appropriate clothing is important as are firm handshakes, eye contact, and good posture. People can often be engaged in conversation when you ask them about something they have done or are associated with. It would therefore behoove you to know something about them or their organization before introducing yourself. Use this knowledge to create conversation. People will speak more readily about institutional issues than personal issues, so start with requests for information or observations about their organization before moving to questions that are more personally professional. Their personal advice may have to wait until another meeting. During the conversation, find cues that allow you to remember their name for next time.

The key to networking is the exchange process. In other words, be useful to others as others are useful to you. Remember to share ideas, offer advice when asked, and provide potential contacts for other people. If you are an undergraduate student, it does not mean that you have little to add. Professionals are always interested in your education, aspirations, and impressions of their organization. Keep in mind that professionals pay good money to attend conferences, and time spent networking should be worth it. When engaged in conversation, listen carefully. If you are stuck for a reply, seek clarification of the comment to buy yourself some time. Don't be afraid to ask questions; this not only demonstrates your interest, but can also help by gathering additional information. If the person seems like a valuable contact by the end of the conversation, request a business card and offer your card too (undergraduate students should have business cards for these occasions).

Once you have made contact, you need to continue to build and maintain them. Make sure that you keep business cards and professional addresses in an organized folder that is regularly updated and organized. Not only should you update your professional address book, but you also should periodically reassess your needs as your priorities and interests change. Consciously make an effort to maintain networks by calling them periodically, sending cards on special occasions, meeting for lunch, or simply dropping a line to say hello. The best way to eliminate the feelings of fakeness is to send the contact an article or resource that has interest for him or her. The most successful networking rests on the premise of sharing. Therefore, sharing information with peers and colleagues is paramount for effective networking. Finally, you need to join and become active in the professional organizations that matter to you. By working with these organizations, you become more professionally connected.

Sports Tourism International Council (STIC)

Professional Organizations

International Headquarters
P.O. Box 5580-Station "F"
Ottawa, Canada K2C #m1
Fax/Phone: 1.613.226.9447
Email: stic@winning.com

The purpose of this organization is to establish a professional association for sports tourism, promote sports tourism research, and to link sports and tourism organizations by establishing and creating

- A research unit for sport tourism
- A database for sport tourism research and application
- An annual conference for the presentation of research and information
- *Journal of Sport Tourism* to disseminate knowledge about sport tourism
- Training and academic programs that lead to certificates, diplomas, and degrees in sport tourism.

SMAANZ (Sport Management Association of Australia and New Zealand

http//132.234.58.200/services.smaanz/SMAANZ.HTM

SMAANZ aims to encourage scholarly inquiry into sport management-related research and to provide the opportunity to present results from this research. This is achieved through an annual conference and a forthcoming refereed journal.

European Society for Sport Management (EASM)

EASM secretariat

c/o ISEF viuzzo di gattaia 9, 50125 Firenze Italy

Email: easm@cesit1.unifi.it

Fax: 39.55.24.17.99

EASM is an independent association for individuals or members representing associations involved in or interested in sport management. The association aims to promote, stimulate, and encourage studies, research, and scholarly writing and professional development in the field of sport management.

Indian Association of Sport Management (IASM)

Secretary General

Department of Physical Education

Mahatma Gandi University, Kottayam - 1

India 686 001

Phone 091.481.560511

Fax: 0091.481.564279

IASM is the only sports management organization in India. It works towards the promotion of quality sports management in India through sports administrators, educators, coaches, and sports people.

Korean Sport Management Association

Korea Sport Marketing Institute (KISM)

P.O. Box 23

Seocho Post Office

Seoul, Korea

Phone 82.335.34.5209

Fax 82.335.33.5450

North American Society for Sport Management (NASSM)

NASSM is the professional association that governs sport management in Canada and the United States. Its purpose is to promote, stimulate, and encourage study, research, scholarly writing and professional development in the area of sport management—both theoretical and applied aspects.

NASSM concerns itself with such diverse issues in sport management as sport marketing, future directions of management, competencies, leadership, sports and the law, human relations management, facility management, organizational structures, fund-raising, and conflict resolution all as they apply to sport. <www.unb.ca/SportManagement/index.htm>

Travel and Tourism Research Association (TTRA)

TTRA is an organization of providers and users of travel and tourism research that serves as a primary resource to the travel and tourism industry <www.ttra.com>

Bicycle Touring Companies

Adventure Cycling Association
(406) 721-1776

Backcountry
(800) 575-1540

Backroads
(800) 462-1540

Bicycle Adventures
(800) 443-6060

Butterfield & Robinson
(800) 678-1147

Cycle America
(800) 245-3263

French Louisiana Bike Tours
(800) 346-7989

Michigan Bicycle Touring
(616) 263-5885

Timberline Bicycle Tours
(303) 759-3804

Vermont Bicycle Touring
(802) 453-4811

Source: "Travel Weekly" 12/4/97 p. 23

Golf Tour Operators

Adventures in Golf— Hamilton Travel Service
(603) 882-8367

Arizona Golf & Leisure
gst@aol.com

Carolina Golf Vacations
www.carolinagolfvacation.com

Classic Golf and Leisure
(619) 722-2563

Connoisseur Golf
connoiseur-golf@compuserve.com

Dylan's Irish and Scottish Golf
(412) 421-4276

GOGO Worldwide Vacations
(201) 934-3500

Golf International
(212) 986-9176

Golfpac Inc.
golfpacinc@aol.com

GolfTrips
peggy5678@aol.com

Grasshopper Golf Tours
(630) 858-1660

Intergolf
intergolf@golftravel.com

ITC Golf Tours
(562) 595-6905

Jerry Quinlan's Celtic Golf
celticgolf@aol.com.

Owenoak International
psgv@aol.com

Palm Springs Golf Vacations
(760) 346-3331

Perrygolf
perrygolf@golftravel.com.

PGA Travel
pgatravel@hgc.travelinc.com

Quinlan Tours-Distinctive Irish Vacations
(609) 884-3462

RoundBall Golf Tours
(817) 459-4653

SGH Golf
sghgolf@cinti.net

Showcase Ireland
ireland@naplesnet.com

Spanish Golf Adventures
info@spanishgolf.com

Sportours
www.sporttours.com

Sportstours
(305) 535-0007

Taurus Tours
taurusev@gte.net

Ultra Adventure Tours
ultratours@ttlc.net

Value Golf Vacations
(212) 986-0393

Wide World of Golf
(408) 624-6667
WWofG@aol.com

Ski Tour Operators

Adventure Tours USA
(214) 360-5050

Adventures on Skis
(413) 568-2855

Alta Tours
(415) 777-1307

Angersbach International Tours
(732) 223-0303

Any Mountain Tours
(703) 378-2SKI

Aspen Ski Tours Inc.
(970) 925-9500

Backroads
(510) 527-1555

BET Tours
(305) 385-8400

Canadian Mountain Holidays, Inc.
(403) 762-7100

Central Holidays
(201) 798-5777

Classic Holiday
(503) 668-3508

Colorado Ski Holidays, Inc.
(719) 534-0990

DER Travel Services
(847) 692-4141

Esprit Tours
(302) 792-3200

Friendly Holidays
(516) 358-1200

Gogo Worldwide Travel
(201) 265-0400

Meier's International L.L.C.
(310) 215-1980

Moguls Ski and Snowboard Tours
(303) 440-7921

Mount Snow Vermont Tours
(802) 464-2076

Mountain Vacations
(800) 775-5252

Off The Beaten Path
(406) 586-1311

RMA Tours
(303) 759-4600

Santa Fe Accommodations
(505) 988-3400

Ski Connections
(916) 582-1892

Ski Vacation Planner
(201) 801-0028

Sportours
(818) 553-3333

TransGlobal Vacations
(612) 948-8000

Colorado International Ski Tours
(719) 471-0222

Continental Vacations
(281) 872-6620

Eastern Light Getaways
(215) 633-6100

Euro Lloyd Tours
(516) 794-1253

Future Tours
(561) 750-1100

Holidaze Ski Tours
(908) 280-1120

Midwest Express Vacations
(414) 934-3434

Morris Travel
(801) 483-6107

Mountain Tours
(203) 259-0178

Northwest World Vacations
(800) 727-1111

Preferred Holidays
(954) 359-7000

Royal Northwest Holidays
(206) 448-9092

Schwartz Tours
(206) 822-6655

Ski Pak
(206) 747-9901

Snow Tours
(201) 348-2244

Tradesco Tours
(310) 649-5808

Travel Organizers
(303) 771-1173

United Vacations
(800) 699-6122,
(800) 328-6877

US Airways Vacations
(800) 544-7733,
(800) 455-0123

Wanderweg Holidays
(609) 321-1040

World of Vacations
(416) 620-8687

**Major League
Baseball
Franchises**

American League

Anaheim Angels
(714) 940-2000

Baltimore Orioles
(410) 685-9800

Boston Red Sox
(617) 267-9440

Chicago White Sox
(312) 674-1000

Cleveland Indians
(216) 420-4200

Detroit Tigers
(313) 962-4000

Kansas City Royals
(816) 921-2200

Minnesota Twins
(612) 375-1366

New York Yankees
(718) 293-4300

Oakland Athletics
(510) 638-4900

Seattle Mariners
(206) 628-3555

Tampa Bay Devil Rays
(813) 825-3137

Texas Rangers
(817) 273-5222

Toronto Blue Jays
(416) 341-1000

National League

Arizona Diamondbacks
(602) 514-8500

Atlanta Braves
(404) 522-7630

Chicago Cubs
(773) 404-2827

Cincinnati Reds
(513) 421-4510

Colorado Rockies
(303) 292-0200

Florida Marlins
(305) 626-7400

Houston Astros
(713) 404-2827

Los Angeles Dodgers
(213) 224-1500

Milwaukee Brewers
(414) 933-4114

Montreal Expos
(514) 253-3434

New York Mets
(718) 507-6387

Philadelphia Phillies
(215) 463-6000

Pittsburgh Pirates
(412) 323-5000

St. Louis Cardinals
(314) 421-3060

San Diego Padres
(619) 283-4494

San Francisco Giants
(415) 468-3700

Source: Travel Weekly, 6/6/98, p. 37.

NBA Franchises

Atlanta Hawks
One CNN Center
South Tower, #405
Atlanta, GA 30303

Boston Celtics
151 Merrimac St., 5th Floor
Boston, MA 02114

Charlotte Hornets
100 Hive Drive
Charlotte, NC 28217
Chicago, IL 60612

Chicago Bulls
United Center
1901 Madison

Cleveland Cavaliers
Gund Arena
100 Gateway Plaza
Cleveland, OH 44115

Dallas Mavericks
Reunion Arena
777 Sports St.
Dallas, TX 75207

Denver Nuggets
1635 Clay St.
Box 4658
Denver, CO 80204-0658

Detroit Pistons
The Palace of Auburn Hills
Two Championship Drive
Auburn Hills, MI 48057

Golden State Warriors
1221 Broadway, 20th Floor
Oakland, CA 94612

Houston Rockets
Two Greenway Plaza, #400
Houston, TX 77277

Indiana Pacers
300 E. Market St.
Indianapolis, IN 46204
Los Angeles, CA 90037

Los Angeles Clippers
Los Angeles Sports Arena
3939 Figueroa

Los Angeles Lakers
Great Western Forum
3900 W. Manchester Blvd.
Inglewood, CA 90305

Miami Heat
One Southeastern Third Ave.
Suite 2300
Miami, FL 33131

Milwaukee Bucks
1001 Fourth St.
Milwaukee, WI 53203-1312

Minnesota Timberwolves
600 First Ave. North
Minneapolis, MN 55403

New Jersey Nets
405 Murray Hill Parkway
East Rutherford, NJ 07073

New York Knicks
Madison Square Garden
2 Pennsylvania Plaza
New York, NY 10121

Orlando Magic
One Magic Place
Orlando, FL 32801

Philadelphia 76ers
Veterans Stadium
Box 25040
Philadelphia, PA 19147-0240

Phoenix Suns
Phoenix Suns Plaza
201 E. Jefferson
Phoenix, AZ 85004

NFL Franchises

Arizona Cardinals
(602) 379-0101

Atlanta Falcons
(770) 945-1111

Baltimore Ravens
(410) 654-6200

Buffalo Bills
(716) 648-1800

Carolina Panthers
(704) 358-7000

Chicago Bears
(847) 295-6600

Cincinnati Bengals
(513) 621-3550

Dallas Cowboys
(214) 556-9000

Denver Broncos
(303) 649-9000

Detroit Lions
(313) 335-4131

Green Bay Packers
(414) 496-5700

Indianapolis Colts
(317) 297-2658

Jacksonville Jaguars
(904) 633-6000

Kansas City Chiefs
(816) 924-9300

Miami Dolphins
(954) 452-7000

Minnesota Vikings
(612) 828-6500

New England Patriots
(508) 543-8200

New Orleans Saints
(504) 733-0255

New York Giants
(201) 935-8111

New York Jets
(516) 538-6600

Oakland Raiders
(510) 864-5000

Philadelphia Eagles
(215) 463-2500

Pittsburgh Steelers
(412) 323-1200

St. Louis Rams
(314) 982-7267

San Diego Chargers
(619) 280-2111

San Francisco 49ers
(408) 562-4949

Seattle Seahawks
(206) 827-9777

Tampa Bay Buccaneers
(813) 870-2700

Tennessee Oilers
(888) 313-TEAM

Washington Redskins
(703) 478-8900

Source: Travel Weekly, 8/27/97 p. 13.

NHL Franchises

Mighty Ducks of Anaheim
(714) 704-2700

Boston Bruins
(617) 624-1050

Buffalo Sabres
(716) 855-4100

Carolina Hurricanes
(919) 467-7825

Calgary Flames
(403) 777-2177

Chicago Blackhawks
(312) 455-7000

Colorado Avalanche
(303) 893-6700

Dallas Stars
(972) 868-2890

Detroit Red Wings
(313) 396-7544

Edmonton Oilers
(403) 474-8561

Florida Panthers
(954) 768-1900

Los Angeles Kings
(310) 419-3160

Montreal Canadiens
(514) 932-2582

New Jersey Devils
(201) 935-6050

New York Islanders
(516) 794-4100

New York Rangers
(212) 456-6000

Ottawa Senators
(613) 599-0250

Philadelphia Flyers
(215) 465-4500

Phoenix Coyotes
(602) 379-2800

Pittsburgh Penguins
(412) 642-1800

St. Louis Blues
(314) 622-2500

San Jose Sharks
(408) 287-7070

Tampa Bay Lightning
(813) 229-2658

Toronto Maple Leafs
(416) 977-1641

Vancouver Canucks
(604) 899-4600

Washington Capitals
(301) 386-7000

Source: Travel Weekly, 10/9/97, p. 21.

Chapter 9

Issues in Sport Tourism

Questions

1. What are the reasons for prevalence of professional sport franchise relocations in North America?
2. What sport tourism issues surround the trend of legalized gambling expansion in the United States?
3. In what ways, if any, has the commercialization of sport detracted from the sport tourism experience?

Introduction

This chapter explores several issues facing the sport tourism industry, including sport facility financing, sport gambling, and over-commercialization of sport. Before discussing these trends, it is necessary to describe the relationship between trends and issues. *Trends* are patterns of human behavior, and *issues* are situations arising from trends. Fads are also patterns of behavior but are contrived, short-lived, and often driven by product manufacturers and marketers.

Another characteristic of issues is that there are often many interpretations or sides of the issue, its causes, impacts, and solutions. Issues are perceived negatively by some, positively by some, and as being of little consequence by others. There is a lack of consensus in solving the issue.

Political, financial, social, historical, and cultural factors often influence the extent of the issue. Finally, for a problem to warrant the issue "status," others must be aware of the its side effects. Below are several examples of sport tourism trends and their related issues.

Trend	Related Issue
Urban stadium development	Local tax increases
Team free agency	Loss of fan identification/loyalty
Gambling	Social costs of compulsive gambling
Promotional licensing	Black market sales
Event sponsorship	Alcohol/tobacco ads

In 1994, over half of the 99 major teams based in the United States had either moved into a new arena or stadium or had plans to build one, most with some public financial support. National Football League (NFL) teams have been the most mobile in the past decade as owners search for more lucrative stadium deals. Is a professional sport franchise a good investment for a city?

Professional sports in North America are experiencing an unprecedented building boom. In 1995, cities and states issued over $500 million dollars in bonds to build new sport facilities. Facilitating this growth in sport facility development is the surge in sport team free agency, as owners are willing to relocate their teams in search of better deals and newer stadiums.

Turco and Ostrosky (1997) chronicled the sport team free agency phenomenon:

> In (American) football, the Colts abandoned Baltimore for Indianapolis in the late 1980's to start the movement of teams to new cities. Since then, the Oakland Raiders have moved to Los Angeles and back again; the St. Louis Cardinals are in Arizona; the New York Giants play in New Jersey; the L.A. Rams are now in St. Louis; the Cleveland Browns have become the Baltimore Ravens; and, the Seattle Seahawks may migrate south to L.A. (p. 101)

They note that prior to 1980, NFL teams did not relocate to other cities.

The NFL's revenue-sharing system is one contributing factor to the team free-agency phenomenon. The NFL divides all television revenues equally among its franchises, including play-off games. Forty percent of ticket receipts go to visiting teams, and merchandising profits are split evenly. To be profitable and competitive on the playing field, many NFL team owners have tapped into unshared income streams, including skybox construction, parking, scoreboard and stadium advertising, personal seat licenses, and concession revenues. Among owners with teams playing in stadiums void of these revenue-generating options, several have approached their local leaders about building a new stadium or renovating the existing facility with public tax support. Because league teams compete in publicly and privately financed facilities, the teams playing in publicly supported facilities have a clear advantage. With less capital tied to debt retirement, teams with publicly financed facilities may use revenues to hire more talented free-agent players. However, having the biggest payroll does not guarantee success on the field.

Owners seeking a new facility with taxpayer dollars claim they want "an even playing field" compared with revenue-generating facilities of other owners. However, critics argue that "the grass will always be greener" in the next stadium built, and owners will again set higher requirements for stadium deals (e.g., parking revenues, lower lease fees, more luxury suites). Owners in other professional sport leagues have requested public assistance with stadium financing. In Chicago, the owner of Major League Baseball's White Sox put pressure on the city by contemplating a move to St. Petersburg. The state and city agreed to help build a new $185-million Comiskey Park.

Many urban officials believe that sport means big business. U.S cities will spend nearly $6 billion for sport stadium development before 2000 (Osterland, 1995). City officials from Milwaukee to Miami have embraced the notion that stadiums and commercial sport are essential in projecting a world-class image. Stadium advocates claim that the image and respectability imparted by professional sport are substantiated by the economic impact of sport. The respectability comes not from having the team's players living in the community per se, but that a professional sport franchise signifies to others that the city is "major league."

Cities in their desire to retain or attract a commercial sports franchise find they have to accommodate or provide for that which teams identify as critical sources of revenue. Civic leaders in some cities believe that new stadiums are essential to retain or acquire at least a professional sport franchise. In the early 1990s, owners of the Cleveland Browns and Houston Oilers gave their respective cities an ultimatum: "Either build a new stadium, or I will move the team to another city." Both cities denied the owners' requests. The Browns moved to Baltimore in 1996, and the Oilers moved to Tennessee. Both owners received new stadiums for their teams.

Cities that have successfully lured sport teams away from other cities anticipate the increased economic activity (and subsequent tax revenues) from sport consumers will offset the costs of the stadium deal. Sport supporters contend that suburbanites and other outsiders will spend their money near the stadium or arena and boost the economy, shifting an urban area's stagnant economic base to an emerging growth sector—tourism.

Not everyone is convinced that professional sport benefits a community and is worthy of taxpayer support. After three referenda failed to produce public support for a new stadium, the owner of the NFL Miami Dolphins decided to build his own. Stadium operating deficits in Pontiac, Michigan, and New Orleans, coupled with poor team win-loss records, have galvanized taxpayer resistance. Residents in San Francisco, Miami, and Chicago have opposed public-financed stadium referenda to build new stadiums.

In light of the footloose sport franchise environment that now prevails, several questions warrant investigation. Is a professional football franchise a good public investment for a city? What is the city's financial return on investment (ROI) on a football stadium?

The "life expectancy" of a stadium is often determined by the sport franchise owner using the facility. A new stadium is also no guarantee that a sport franchise will not move. The Detroit Lions of the NFL announced that they will leave the 21-year-old Pontiac Silverdome for a new stadium to be built in Detroit (Turco & Ostrosky, 1997). Pittsburgh built two professional sports facilities, one for football and one for baseball, to replace Riverfront Stadium, built in the 1970s (Nelson, 1996).

Reported impacts of sport franchises on their host economies have varied widely, calling into question the validity of such findings. Granted, inaccurate assumptions, gross procedural errors, and misapplication of multipliers have occurred by researchers in estimating the impacts of sport on host economies. Principles, methods, and data requirements to accurately measure the economic impact of sport tourism on the host area are described in Chapter 3.

From an economic impact modeling perspective, nonresident expenditures are made by those who would not have come to the city had the team not been playing, including players, coaches, staff of visiting teams, league representatives, officials, and media personnel. Care must be taken to measure only visitor expenditures that would not have occurred in the absence of the team. Impacts on an economy attributable to a sport franchise also may include operating personnel wages and other expenditures made locally (e.g., promotions, commodities). Many have rightfully criticized the impacts of sport fran-

Sport Tour: Traveling With the NFL Rams

One of the best sport franchise deals involved the Los Angeles Rams and the people of St. Louis, Missouri. Two NFL teams moved out of Los Angeles in 1995, the Raiders to Oakland (attracted by $100 million in stadium renovation) and the Rams to St. Louis (which built a $260-million domed stadium). The deal that brought the Rams back to St. Louis gave the team owners $20 million annually in stadium revenue, including all earnings from 120 luxury suites, all concession revenues, and 75% of stadium advertising revenues, or 90% when advertising revenues total $6 million or more. Prices for luxury suites range from $47,500 to $75,000, depending upon size and location. The deal also included a new $20 million practice facility and $60 million from personal seat licenses (PSLs), which require fans to pay as much as $4,500 to guarantee the right to buy season tickets for $360 (Phares, 1995). Ten years earlier, St. Louis tried to prevent the NFL Cardinals from moving to Phoenix by offering to build a new stadium for an estimated $111 million (Crothers, 1995). The new domed stadium near downtown St. Louis will be paid for by taxpayers until the year 2022. The city and county each pay $6 million per year, and the state of Missouri pays $12 million. Approximately $4.2 million from the proceeds of PSL sales went for actual stadium construction.

chises and stadium deals on urban economies. Further, some have suggested that deals to attract/retain franchises are politically motivated, and that such influence has even tainted the validity of the economic impact research used to "sell the deal" to the public.

Contrary to Baade's argument (1996), a sport franchise can be a good deal for the host economy, under certain circumstances. First, it must induce large net increases in spending from sources outside the designated economy. Examples of this may include the following:

1. Team personnel, headquarters, practice and preseason training facilities reside within the host economy.

2. The playing facility is multipurpose with the ability to host longer events (e.g., Super Bowl, NCAA Men's Basketball Final Four, NBA All-Star Game).

3. The team attracts peripheral business development (e.g., lodging accommodations, eating and drinking places, retail shops).

To be competitive with others as a host site for large-scale sporting events such as the Olympic Games or World Cup, a community must possess, at a minimum, direct air and ground transportation. an adequate number and variety of lodging accommodations, and exhibition facilities. Without a suitable sport facility and infrastructure, the community would not even be considered. Domes are the fashion in stadium design, and dome stadium construction costs are substantial. Every domed stadium in the United States has been built with public funds.

Another side to the sport-tourism ROI equation is similar to the "lost opportunity cost" point of contention often made by sport stadium critics. Economic impact studies essentially seek to determine what would be missed in terms of nonresident direct expenditures had the team in question vacated the local economy. However, resident income retention is equally important to an economy. Ascertaining the amount of resident income leaked from an economy as a result of their attendance at a game in another city also involves opportunity-cost projection. If the Rams had not come to St. Louis, how much income would have gone to Kansas City or Chicago with football fans from St. Louis?

Stadium financing is a complex arrangement, often involving private investments, state, county and city taxes, and revenues from ticket sales. In the short run, spending by local sports fans does not represent an increase in spending on leisure activities, but is merely a diversion of leisure dollars from other activities. People have only so much to spend on entertainment. Spending at home games comes out of personal income that otherwise would have gone for movie or theater tickets, concerts, museums, or theme parks. However, local spending can be counted if it would have been made outside the economy had not the sport team been playing.

Baade (1994) suggests that public funding of professional sport stadiums is a poor investment and that public investments would realize higher return for other purposes: "Spent differently, either by public officials on different public services or by private citizens who are not taxed to subsidize sports, these large sums of money may contribute more to an area's growth" (p. 12). In light of the present building boom, it appears that public support for high-visibility development projects like stadiums and arenas is greater than for many alternatives.

> The notion of a community elevating its image as a "major league sport city" is one often met with little regard by opponents to sport development. Yet, sport championship organizers like the NCAA, World Cup, and NFL, go with a winner, and select a city based on its successful track-record for hosting large-scale events.
>
> They conclude that decisions on the financial ROI of a professional sport franchise should be made on a case-by-case basis rather than in aggregate. "As different as the teams' personnel, so too are the local economies, stadium deals, and impact variables" (p. 109).

Previous research on sport franchise recruitment and retention by communities has been primarily quantitative. Many qualitative impacts of sport do exist for the host community. For example, a sport franchise is related to the "image" of a city, both by outsiders and by residents. Turco and Ostrosky (1997) ask, "At what cost, image?"

Sport Gambling

The U.S. gambling industry realized unprecedented growth in the 1990s. By the start of the new millennium, some form of legalized gambling will exist in every state, except Hawaii and Utah. Approximately 92 million visits to casinos were made in 1993, twice the number of visits made in 1990, placing casino-going ahead of other leisure experiences, such as attending professional baseball games and concerts. It is expected that the amount wagered on legal gambling in America will rise to $500 billion by the year 2000.

Illinois is one of several states where riverboat casinos are permitted. In 1995, riverboat gambling revenues generated $140 million in state and local tax revenue, created 8,800 jobs, and generated $158 million in employee wages. It is clear that big money surrounds the gambling industry, but not all gamblers are wealthy.

Opponents of legalized gambling claim that it is regressive in nature; the poor spend a disproportionate amount of their income on gambling than the rich or middle class. In their study of poor gamblers, Turco, Riley and Lee (1999) reported that "the poor are more likely to spend two-and-a-half times the percentage of their income on gambling as the middle class . . . gambling is the only 'investment' many of the working poor think they can afford." In tough times, middle- and upper-class folk stopped playing the lotteries, but poor urban dwellers kept right on playing.

To diversify and expand their consumer markets, Las Vegas and Atlantic City have hosted many sporting events. Boxing matches have been the preferred sport over the years, but other events, including golf, automobile racing, strongest man competition, and rodeo, have been staged.

> Casinos are marketed by operators and perceived by consumers as romantic, glamorous, and exciting. They attempt to create a "high-roller," VIP image for their consumers. Casinos offer a sensory explosion of sounds, colors, lights, and images that create a hypnotic atmosphere for gamblers. Video gambling and slot machines offer players immediate gratification and feedback. They are easy to understand, unlike deciphering horse race betting sheets. Slot machine players tend to be lower educated, have lower income, and be older than those who participate in other forms of gambling.

There are several management considerations associated with casinos that affect the host community's tourism industry. Casino operations are more labor-intensive than other properties because of their 24-hour activity, a factor that drives operating costs up. Several other problems unique to the gaming industry include the following:

1. More transient labor

2. Round-the-clock (24-hour) operations

3. Increased security requirements

4. Control of undesirables and pathological consumers

5. Entertainment management

6. Gaming management

Lodging and/or food and beverages are typically priced cheaply or offered complimentarily as incentives to draw and retain customers, rather than priced to make profits. This strategy undermines competing accommodation businesses from capitalizing on tourist volume associated with sport gambling.

Atlantic City, New Jersey vs. Las Vegas, Nevada

Atlantic City, New Jersey, attracts approximately 30 million people each year. The average length of stay for a visitor is less than one day. By comparison, visitors stay in Las Vegas an average of 4.3 days. Atlantic City has attempted to position itself as a gambling city, whereas Las Vegas is marketing itself as a complete family destination.

Las Vegas has over 100,000 hotel rooms, with an average occupancy rate of 85%, 20% higher than the nationwide average. It hosts 500 conventions annually that average over 2,000 delegates. The combination business/pleasure traveler spends on average $810 per trip and accounts for 42% of Las Vegas occupancy.

Approximately 60 million people live within a day's drive of Atlantic City, and the automobile is most gamblers' primary form of transportation. Over 12 million of the 30 million annual visitors arrive on junket buses and stay an average of 6 hours. Away from the famous Boardwalk, by the late 1990s, water and sewer systems were deteriorated, streets in poor condition and of insufficient size to accommodate increased traffic, buildings abandoned, and a majority of the city's businesses closed. Major airlines are reluctant to schedule many flights to Atlantic City until sufficient convention facilities are built.

Racing

The thoroughbred horse-racing industry contributes $500 billion annually to the U.S. economy, with owners alone accounting for $13 billion in annual investments and maintenance expenditures. Dog racing appeals to some sport gamblers because it has a faster turnover than horses (more races per hour). Avid dog-racing fans revel in the challenge of picking a winner and claim that the odds in dog racing are more favorable than in horse racing.

Dog racing is also a popular sport tourism option because it affords more people with opportunities for direct involvement. Dogs require smaller overhead costs for maintenance in comparison to horses, creating greater access for people to assume ownership and investment in the sport. These advantages over horse racing have not been enough to save the many dog-racing tracks in Wisconsin built in the 1990s from closing or filing bankruptcy.

To compensate for some of their competitive disadvantages with other gambling options, horse-racing marketers have attempted to position their product as having a sense of history, tradition, socialization, celebration, pageantry, and aesthetic beauty. The human element associated with horse racing (jockeys) has caused controversy, as some riders have been known to throw a race for illegal financial gain. The lengthy time between horse races and slower event pace has caused some race tracks to install video simulcasts of other races and request that video games and slot machines be authorized.

Future of Sport Gambling

Opposition to gambling will continue to be more vocal, organized, and "politically" astute. Coalitions against gambling in Nebraska have encouraged voters on three separate occasions to reject referenda calling for casinos.

In spite of more organized opposition, people will continue to gamble, and more gambling outlets will emerge. Legalized pro and college sport betting with distribution points similar to off-track betting parlors are envisaged. In the future, it is anticipated that alternative sports betting (pari-mutuel) will increase in popularity, particularly in bicycle racing and snowmobile racing. Finally, the extent to which sport gambling via the Internet will affect tourism visitation is unknown at this point. On one hand, it may stimulate more interest in gambling and subsequent visitation at sport venues. Conversely, Internet sport gambling may supplant in-person visitation and contribute to reduced tourism volume.

Discussion Questions— Sport Gambling

1. Several issues surround sport betting. What are the economic costs and benefits resulting from legalized gambling? Social costs and benefits?

2. Does government have a responsibility to rectify and pay for the social costs attributed to compulsive gambling? Should government be "in the business" of authorizing gambling? Why or why not?

Overcommercialization of Sport   One has only to view a professional automobile race, tennis match, or basketball game and count the numerous corporate names and logos appearing on the participants and signs in the stadiums to agree that the use of sponsor visibility in sport is widespread (Mullin, Hardy, & Sutton, 1993). Prior to the 1990s, most dasher boards surrounding professional hockey rinks were barren. Today they are littered with advertisements. From the sporting event organizer's perspective, merchandise sales, sponsorship and advertising signage, and concession items sales are major revenue sources.

Increasingly, sport tourism experiences that once were free are now being produced, "packaged," and sold to consumers. For example, use permits are now required to cross country ski in some U.S. Forest Service areas. Admission to the World Series of Little League Baseball was once free of charge. Today paid admission tickets are required, and concessions and souvenirs items are promoted and sold. The growth in sport sponsorship has contributed to commercialization of sport, as companies seek ways to entice spectators to try their products. Licensed sport merchandise and memorabilia are sold at ballparks, in stores, and online. Stadiums are littered with billboards, signs, and other commercial messages. Advertising exists almost everywhere in sport—even in the restrooms! The commercialization of sport tourism may lead some consumers to seek attractions that are pure, and void of such commercial intrusions.

The nature of the Kodak Albuquerque International Balloon Fiesta permits considerable promotional visibility and numerous sponsorship exposures. Many balloons prominently feature corporate logos on the balloon envelope. Considering the size of the balloons, corporate images on inflated balloons may be as large as 50' × 50', making the promotion a "floating billboard." Some balloons are shaped in the form of a corporation's product (e.g., Pepsi can, Burger King burger, Famous Footwear athletic shoe) or prominent icon (e.g., Kellogg's Tony the Tiger, Klondike's polar bear). Balloons ascend each morning of the event and during four shows at dusk.

Those who argue that sport is overcommercialized point to the athletes' attire, replete with sponsor logos; network television requirements for game timeouts; and mass-merchandising opportunities. They contend that sport authenticity has been compromised for the sake of financial gain. Other commercial examples include made-for-television events, ESPN's X-Games and golf's Skins Game. What effects, if any, do these commercial operations have on spectators' perceptions of the sport tourism experience? Has sport reached the point of commercial saturation? Is there a consumer backlash as a result of increased commercialization in sport?

---

1. In what ways do sport tourism consumers and/or suppliers contribute to commercialization?

2. Select an actual sport tourism attraction with both cultural and historic significance. Describe (in detail) how the authenticity of the attraction has been maintained (or compromised).

Discussion Questions— Sport Commercialization

Host-Guest Interactions

The final issue covered in this chapter involves conflicts that may arise from sport tourists visiting destinations with less than receptive residents. Much has been written about the irritants that tourists cause, as perceived by residents (Doxey, 1975). Not all sport tourists are wanted or welcomed. Consider the many black residents of Atlanta's central district whose homes, churches, and businesses were displaced by construction of facilities for the 1996 Summer Olympics. Their reaction to the event was not one of euphoria but of resentment.

During the spring, the greater Phoenix, Arizona, area is one of the most popular regions in the United States in which to watch professional baseball exhibition games. Thousands of older adults from the Northeast and Midwest flock, often in recreational vehicles, to the area in the

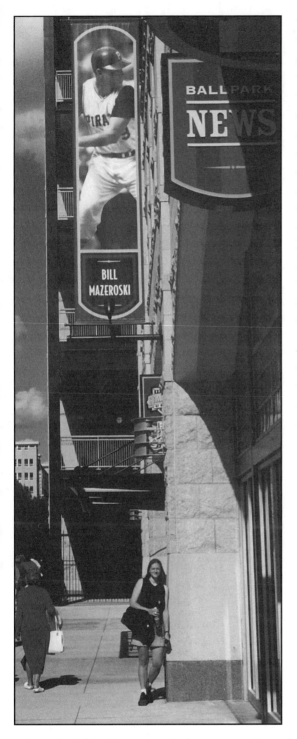

Local residents may not always react positively to the influx of sport tourists in their area.

Photo reprinted by permission
of Jackie Kurkowski.

winter to escape the cold weather and stay to watch the games. Once the regular baseball season begins and the weather becomes mild, they return to their homes. These sport tourists have been labeled "snowbirds" because of their migratory patterns. Healthcare professionals in the greater Phoenix area have been concerned about the available facilities and costs to provide medical care for these visitors, most of whom are in their sixties. In Scottsdale, Arizona, local officials considered allocating a portion of the lodging tax for healthcare subsidization. One reason that lodging taxes are acceptable to politicians and their constituents is that it shifts some of the financial burden for public goods and services on the visitors.

As discussed in Chapter 5, the importance of community involvement in the sport tourism event planning process cannot be overemphasized if good host-guest relations are to be achieved.

Chapter 10

Future Directions in Sport Tourism

Questions

1. How are trends distinguished from fads?
2. What impacts will technological advances have on sport tourism?
3. How would adverse environmental conditions affect the future of participatory sport tourism?

In the United States, 38% of adults attended an organized sports event, competition, or tournament between 1993–1998, as either a spectator or a participant. These adults, estimated at over 75.3 million, had traveled more than 50 miles one way for the events. 70% of these people had traveled for sports within the last year of the survey period. 84% were spectators at the sporting events and 50% of all the travel was oriented toward professional sports. Just over 20% traveled to see children's porting events and 18% made special purchases of sporting equipment or clothes before leaving home.*

As sport becomes more important as economic and cultural phenomena, the relationships between sporting events, venues, and visitors will continue to receive attention from tourism industry segments, trade associations, and host cities. Media coverage of hallmark events such as the Olympic Games, the World Cup, Grand Prix Racing, or a major golf championship expose people to sport in record numbers and stimulate a desire for many to witness the spectacles in person. The tourism industry has already capitalized on some of the regional and national interest in sports competition, and now, through global media channels and Internet communications, sport experiences and events can be marketed globally in an instant. While reaching an international audience instantaneously has its advantages, the sport tourism event marketer must be careful for what she/he wishes. When consumer demand exceeds supply, several negative consequences may arise. Remember the

*Source: www.tia.org/press/093098sports.stm_

Internet and telephone ticketing systems for the World Cup in France that caused safety and public relations nightmares for the organizers?

Although the exact future is uncertain, change in the sport tourism industry is the only certainty. There are more people in the world, more consumers of sport tourism, more travel, more powerful technology, and more sophisticated commercial enterprises offering sport tourism opportunities.

Having placed the caveat that future predictions are merely best guesses, it is worth reviewing the organization of this chapter. It is divided into subtopics that include futures related to demographics, lifestyles, environmental concerns, technology, marketing, and the changing sport tourism marketplace. Although these areas are linked, each possesses unique distinguishing characteristics. For example, in terms of demographics, it is amazing to think that the world's population is growing so rapidly. Does this growth mean there will be more sport tourists and sport participants, or does it mean there will be fewer opportunities to engage in sport because competition for space will be high? The threat of global warming is predicted to alter nature of the destinations that people visit. On the other hand, some scientists think that global warming could have the reverse effect and plunge the world into an ice age. How will these occurrences change sport tourism? Perhaps the most noticeable changes will occur in the marketplace of sport tourism. There will be changes in the way visitors are attracted to events, changes in the types of events promoted and in the way the services are delivered to visitors. These themes will be discussed in greater depth later in this chapter, but first, it is worthwhile to review the differences between trends and fads so that one is not confused with the other. It is also valuable to review the outlook of the travel and tourism phenomenon as predicted by the World Tourism Organization (WTO) and other sources.

Trends vs. Fads

Trends tend to be enduring phenomena whereas fads have a short life span. According to Letscher (1997), fads burst onto the scene, increase rapidly, and then fade when replaced by other activities. With this description in mind, there are some ways to identify trends. These indicators are related to consumer trends rather than trends of natural phenomenon, because sport tourism depends upon consumption. Letscher's largely informs the guidelines below.

- Lifestyle fit—Does the trend fit other lifestyle trends or changes in consumer world? For example, consumers have increasing expectations of convenience when making purchases. For sport tourism products and services to become trends, they must be easily consumable in terms of time and effort. Innovations in travel have made greater convenience possible, but innovation in communication technology will likely provide more convenient consumption in the future.

- Multiple benefits—A consumer trend will have many benefits, so it appeals to more than one consumer segment and offers variety to individuals. Multiple benefits will keep consumers involved for longer periods of time and at higher levels of intensity. It will not be sufficient to offer only sports at sport tourism destinations. There will have to be many attractions for everyone to see and do. Sports fans may be totally engaged by sporting events, but partners, traveling companions, and families may require other activities to attract them to the destinations. Furthermore, the tourism activities will need to be varied for different levels of ability and interest. Essentially, large-scale sports destinations will need to become one-stop shops, offering multiple attractions beyond the major sports attractions.

- Customization—In a world made modern by "McDonaldization" (one size fits all), people are demanding consumable products and services that can be modified or personalized for their individual consumption. Sporting events, activities, and sports destinations will soon fade if they are not adaptable or flexible to individual needs. Sport tourism activities have a greater chance of survival if they customize their services while pushing for more tourists. This is especially true as people change from being gazers at and spectators of sports spectacles to consumers who demand participation in sporting events.

- The influentials—Many potential trends have died because influential leaders have not adopted them. To become a trend, the phenomenon needs to be adopted and championed by an influential group that other consumers will follow. Perhaps the retiring baby boomers will be the future influentials of sport tourism, or it may be the increasing number of women who are interested in sports. Whatever the group, they must be powerful enough to excite other consumers to continue the trend. A prime group of influentials are the media companies that can see the economic benefit of long-term support in particular sporting events. Influential people (or companies) who have an economic stake in sport tourism will be more inclined to keep a sport in front of consumers. Equally and oppositely, they will also be likely to discard a sport that does not realize the envisioned economic gains.

- Unrelated influences—Trends must receive unwitting support from happenings and trends in other areas of life. For example, if society became socially conservative, sports that push the social acceptability envelope would be doomed to failure. A case in point would be the permissive antics of professional wrestlers. An unrelated influence, suggested by Letscher (1997), is the increase of individualism in the world. People are becoming less group and community oriented, and more individualistic. This influence bodes well for individual sporting activities but not for team sports where coordination and cooperation are becoming increasingly difficult. Free-market principles of player free agency and team relocation have lessened the collective identity of some professional sport teams for many spectators.

- Technological dependency—If a sport is dependent upon a particular technological innovation, it will likely fail as a trend. In a world where technology is changing so rapidly, technologically dependent sports are certain to be replaced by other innovations. This thought can be illustrated by using the example of musical reproductive devices. For many years, the only way to listen to music was through vinyl records and record players. However, they were soon replaced by eight track tapes, cassette tapes, compact discs, and recently, digital audio technology. Similarly, a sport can be invented, refined, and die with each technological innovation. Cycling is a good example. With the commercial production of 10-speed bicycles, road cycling became popular, and everyone owned a 10-speed. This caused the demise of the one-speed cycles. Nowadays, 10-speed cycles have faded in the face of innovations that have led to mountain bikes and all-terrain cycles.

- Age-group origin—A sport is likely to be a fad when adopted by a single cohort group. This is especially true for teens. Without involvement from other age-groups, a trend rarely continues. Adopters move into other phases of their lives, and they leave behind many of their favorite activities. The exploratory nature of teens means they will move from one activity to another in quick succession. Adoption by a more stable cohort group will afford a greater chance of becoming a trend as will adoption by several cohort groups.

These indicators are just a few of the ways in which trends and fads can be identified. Other trends that can affect sport tourism are those with a natural origin. Climatic patterns and population growth are two such trends. Before discussing some natural trends in depth, it is worth reviewing the trends of tourism in general. The following section is a review of some tourism organizations around the world.

General Tourism Trends

According to a 1997 report from the World Tourism Organization (WTO), travel will be conducted further from home and at a faster pace than that experienced in the early parts of the 20th century. The WTO is also predicting the advent of commercial travel in space. These predictions are not surprising given the increased accessibility of high-speed travel and the technological innovations that allow people to travel further and faster.

Tourism is the world's largest growth industry. Since 1980, international tourism receipts have grown at an average of 9% each year, and during the same period, visitor arrivals have grown by 4.6% (WTO, 1999).

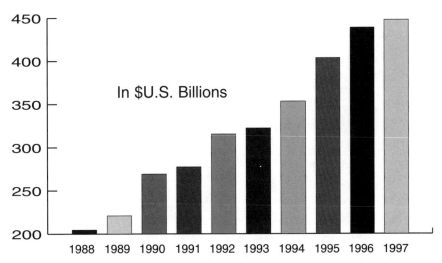

Figure 10.1. Recent Growth Rate in World Tourism Receipts
Source: http://www.tia.org/press/fastfacts6.htm.

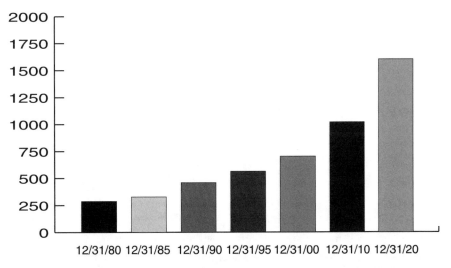

Figure 10.2. Projected International Tourist Arrivals Until 2020

In 2020, the World Travel Organization predicts that 1.6 billion people will visit foreign countries. They will spend more than $US 2 trillion per year or $5 billion per day. This prediction is more than three times the number of people who traveled internationally in 1996, and nearly five times the amount of spending. International travel is an economic and migrational juggernaut. The WTO report predicts that international travel will grow at a rate of 4.3% per year, over the next two decades, with international tourism receipts growing by 6.7% per year. The percentage of long-haul travel will increase from 18% of all international travel in 1995, to 24% in 2020. Possibly the most interesting predictions are the destinations that will become popular destinations by 2020. Some traditional countries will remain popular, but countries without international travel traditions (e.g., China) will rise rapidly as tourist destinations. To note the differences, compare tables 10.1 and 10.2.

Of the top 10 tourist destinations in 1998, 6 were European countries. This is not surprising given the proximity of the European countries and the ease with which visitors can cross international borders. In addition, some European countries enjoy some of the highest living standards in the world and the longest periods of paid vacation time. Therefore, people in these countries have the discretionary income, time, and interest necessary to travel beyond their borders. Another 3 of the top 10 countries are joined at borders also. The United States, Mexico, and Canada all benefit from their immediate proximity to each other and their ability to leverage discretionary income. The aberrant country is China, but it had the highest one-year increase of all countries in 1998.

Table 10.1. Top Ten Tourist Destinations—1998

Rank	Countries	Tourist Arrivals (millions)
1	France	70
2	Spain	47.7
3	United States	47.1
4	Italy	34.8
5	United Kingdom	25.5
6	China	24
7	Mexico	19.3
8	Poland	18.8
9	Canada	18.7
10	Austria	17.2

Source: World Tourism Organization (www.world-tourism.org-newslett/febmar99/1998res.htm)

Table 10.2. Top Ten Tourist Destinations—2020

Rank	Countries	Tourist Arrivals (millions)
1	China	137.1
2	United States	102.4
3	France	93.3
4	Spain	71
5	Hong Kong	59.3
6	Italy	52.9
7	United Kingdom	52.8
8	Mexico	48.9
9	Russian Federation	47.1
10	Czech. Republic	44

Source: World Tourism Organization (www.world-tourism.org-newslett/nov97/travel.htm)

By the year 2020, it is predicted that China will become the number one tourist destination in the world. Although their tourism generation is minuscule at present, the WTO calculates that China will be the fourth largest tourist-generating area by 2020. Other popular destinations will be Russia, Hong Kong, Thailand, Singapore, Indonesia, and South Africa (WTO, 1997). Although the traditionally large-draw destinations remain in the top 10, their ranking will typically fall, especially the European countries. With long-haul travel and a wider array of countries generating travelers, different destinations appear in the list at the expense of Hungary, Poland, and Canada. Entering the top 10 will be the former Soviet Union and Hong Kong. In 2020, Europe will still be a major recipient of tourists, but the Pacific Rim countries, especially those in Asia, will become larger players in the world tourism market. Organizations interested in large audiences will need to reposition their locations and also alter some of their marketing strategies to attract visitors who are not considered today. Clearly, the emerging markets for destinations and tourism-generating areas are the former Communist bloc countries and those on the Pacific Rim, in Asia. In support of this contention, the Korean National Tourist Office (1997) predicts a 10% increase in Asia/Pacific tourism every year for the near future. By 2001, they predict that 20 million Japanese tourists and 10 million Chinese tourists will leave their borders. Outbound tourism from the former Eastern Bloc and Russia will also increase greatly. They further predict that ecotourism and changes from sightseeing to participatory tourism will become prevalent. International tourism will become the largest industry in the world in a short period of time.

The world's tourism industry is already large. If all the people employed by the travel and tourism industry lived in one country, that country would rank 10th in population, just behind Japan. Tourism would have a gross national product of $US 3.5 trillion, ranking second only to the United States. It would also be the world's fastest growing country in terms of population and gross national product (Tom's Tourism Homepage, 1998).

The rest of this chapter is dedicated to the discussion of themes related to the future of sport tourism. The themes take general looks at the future of seemingly natural occurrences and the future of business occurrences. Natural occurrences refer to events in demographics and the environment. Business-related themes delve into technology, marketing, and the sports tourism marketplace.

- Demographic changes in the world and effects on sport tourism

- Behavior and lifestyle changes with regard to sport tourism

- Sport tourism's reaction to environmental change

- Technology and sport tourism

- Changes in sport tourism marketing

- Changes in the sport tourism marketplace

Demographics

Demographics are descriptions of populations in terms of numbers, age distribution, education, racial characteristics, income, education levels, and various other factors. For sport tourism, the study of demographics is important because it will provide some indication about the potential for sports participants and spectators worldwide. Few data describe the "average" sport tourist in demographic terms, so many of the prognostications are speculative. However, according to Delpy (1998), the average U.S. sport tourist looks like the demographic characteristics stated in the list below. Because the United States is a geographically large and relatively affluent country, one would expect sport tourism to occur farther from home than it would for sport tourists in many other countries. Sport tourists from other countries may travel less frequently and spend less money when traveling in comparison to U.S. sport tourists. Indicators do show that U.S. residents will continue to be mainly domestic travelers due to lack of corresponding vacation times among dual-career family members, lack of interest in travelling abroad, and lack of passport ownership.

- Physically active

- Earn more than $45,000 per year

- 18–44 years old

- More educated than the average individual

- Typically travels more than the average individual

Although the average American sport tourist tends to be more affluent than other Americans, only 6% of these people spend more than $2,500 on a typical sports excursion; the majority of sport tourists spend less than $500 (Delpy, 1998). This would tend to suggest that sport tourism is often short in duration and regional in its dispersion. Longer durations and greater distances would require the spending of more money.

The data available on the average sport tourist in the United States suggest that these people engage in physical activity and have large amounts of discretionary income that can be assigned to their sporting passion and to their travel. However, there are contradictory examples. Consider

Year	Population
0	0.3
1000	0.31
1250	0.4
1500	0.5
1750	0.79
1800	0.98
1850	1.26
1900	1.65
1910	1.75
1920	1.86
1930	2.07
1940	2.3
1950	2.25
1960	3.02
1970	3.7
1980	4.45
1990	5.3
1994	5.63
2000	6.23
2025	8.47
2050	10.02
2100	11.19
2150	11.54
2200	11.6

Figure 10.3. World Population Projection Until 2200.

professional football fans in the United States who maintain a very sedentary lifestyle and are derogatorily labeled as "couch potatoes."

The average sport tourist's education level also suggests that he or she is more aware of the opportunities that arise with regard to sport tourism and is able to take advantage of these opportunities when they occur. If extrapolated to the populations of the world, these characteristics severely limit those who can engage in sport tourism. However, the world's people are becoming more affluent and increasingly educated (Population Council, 1999). Increased world affluence and education would suggest a healthy pool of potential travelers to support the growth of sport tourism in the future, although inequalities will persist.

At this time, it is instructive to analyze the population of the world to see what the future may bring. It will be necessary to look at the total population and how it is growing. Then it will be necessary to see where the potential sport tourists may reside in the future. Finally, it will be instructive to review current income levels, age levels, and gender makeup to ascertain the potential growth areas.

The world's population is growing exponentially. Simply stated, it doubles itself in increasingly short intervals. From the inception of humankind, the world did not achieve a population of one billion until around the year 1800. In the next 100 years (approximately 1890), the population reached 1.7 billion people. With the new millennium, the world population will exceed 6 billion individuals (U.S. Census Bureau, 1999) and will continue to grow until it is projected to level off between 11 and 12 billion people (Population Information Network, 1994).

For the tourism entrepreneur, this incredible increase in the world's population may be wonderful news because there will be many potential sport tourists who are ready to travel. For others, this data may be alarming because it invokes thoughts of increased global warming through the overuse of resources, lack of available space to fit people, famine, and other population pathologies. For demographers, politicians, and planners the key question is whether the world can sustain its population or whether some populations will not be able to survive. Even more interesting is that less than 4% of the growth will occur in economically developed nations. With these striking population increases in underdeveloped countries, the economic "haves" will continue to prosper whereas the "have-nots" will struggle to feed their people. Viewing the regions where the population will grow most rapidly also gives an indication of which regions have the most potential in terms of numbers.

By reviewing Table 10.3 it is evident that most of the world's population has resided in Asia/Oceania historically, with no less than 60% of the

Table 10.3. Populations by Regions of the World (millions)

Year	World Total	Europe & USSR	North America	Latin America	Asia & Africa	Oceania
1750	**694**	**144**	**1**	**10**	**100**	**439**
(% of world pop.)	1	0.207	0.001	0.014	0.144	0.633
1900	**1571**	**423**	**81**	**63**	**141**	**863**
(% of world pop.)	1	0.269	0.052	0.04	0.09	0.549
1950	**2520**	**549**	**166**	**166**	**224**	**1416**
(% of world pop.)	1	0.218	0.066	0.066	0.089	0.562
1975	**4077**	**676**	**239**	**320**	**414**	**2427**
(% of world pop.)	1	0.166	0.059	0.078	0.102	0.595
1995	**5716**	**727**	**293**	**482**	**728**	**3487**
(% of world pop.)	1	0.127	0.051	0.084	0.127	0.61

world's total population residing there today. It is not surprising that the World Tourism Organization predicts Asia as the largest growth area for tourism through the year 2020. Also interesting is the fact that the largest tourism-receiving and tourism-generating regions (North America and Europe) made up only 17.8% of the world's population, in 1995. Countries in these two regions were primarily developed nations, and with some exceptions, the majority of the lesser-developed countries were located in the other three regions (Asia, Africa, and Latin America).

Therefore, much of the tourism generated in modern times has come from a very small percentage of the world's population. With the economically developing countries having large sources of potential sport tourists, marketers and sport tourism entrepreneurs will have to focus their efforts here to make their profits. However, in the long term, they will need to widen their focus to include sports and sport tourists from countries in the other three regions. With 90% of world's births taking place in developing countries in 1998 (U.S. Census Bureau, 1999), the population pools in these regions are bountiful for sports tourism entrepreneurs, but it will depend on the future discretionary income of their citizens. Future booms in travel will depend not only on decreased travel cost but also increased income levels, education, and desire to travel for residents of countries where the populations are exploding.

As the tables related to the gross domestic product per capita indicate, the developed nations have significantly more monetary resources per person than do the economically developing nations. The disparity is remarkable. It is also reasonably fair to assume that more people in developed nations will have discretionary money that they can spend on

Table 10.4. Income Per Capita of People in Developed and Developing Nations

Developed Countries		Developing Countries	
Country	Income	Country	Income
Switzerland	$40,746	Brazil	$4,648
Norway	$36,293	Mexico	$3,554
Denmark	$33,387	Thailand	$3,136
Germany	$28,728	Estonia	$2,975
Sweden	$28,546	Russian Federation	$2,974
Singapore	$27,693	Latvia	$2,007
United States	$27,420	Lithuania	$1,510
Belgium	$26,403	Sri Lanka	$771
Netherlands	$25,426	China	$671
Australia	$22,235	India	$375
United Kingdom	$19,847	Kenya	$330
Canada	$19,515	Rwanda	$241

Source: United Nations—Social Indicators, 1999.

sport tourism. Nevertheless, this large disparity in wealth should not deter sport tourism events and entrepreneurs from exploring developing nations as tourist-generating regions and locations for sport tourism. First, these countries are no less interested in sports. Brazil is passionate about soccer, as is India for cricket and the Dominican Republic for baseball. Second, in every country, there are wealthy people who can engage in sport tourism. Third, 96% of the world's population increase will occur in lesser-developed nations (U.S. Census Bureau, 1998).

Of the top 20 tourism-generating nations, only the Russian Federation is included from countries considered to be developing. Germany, the United States and Japan head the list with 50.7 billion, 45.9 billion, and 36.8 billion respectively (Tom's Tourism Homepage, 1997)

Another area of demographics that must be considered carefully is the increasing age of populations in developed countries. Life expectancies have increased 50% since 1950 (Population Council, 1999). Increased life expectancy is due to higher standards of living, better nutrition, and expanded health services. In developed nations, the pyramid age structure has now been replaced with a structure that looks more oblong. Between 1998 and 2025, the number of people in the world 65 years and older will double, whereas the number of people under 15 years of age will increase by only six percent (U.S. Census Bureau, 1998). In developed countries, the older, retired adults will have large discretionary incomes and lots of time to spend freely. They must be made into a viable market segment if sport tourism is to continue to grow. Although older adults are more likely to be spectators, they are also demanding more active tourism pursuits because their health is better than ever before.

The final demographic segment considered in this section is that of women. Although women's salaries and rates of work lag behind those of men, they are now working outside the home more than ever and are slowly increasing their wealth and discretionary income (United Nations, Report on the Beijing Conference, 1998). In developed countries, the economic gap between men and women is closing, and sport entrepreneurs have started to scratch the surface of this powerful market with a variety of sporting opportunities. Twenty years after Title IX in the United States, women's sports are thriving in terms of spectators. The variety of opportunities for participation and the development of professional leagues have increased women's interest. For example, nearly 40% of new golfers in the United States are women, and the number of women who hunt for game has doubled in last 10 years. Women now constitute 15 to 20% of all sports shooters (Delpy, 1998). Other indicators of the increasing markets for women and sport are seen in U.S. collegiate sports. Collegiate women's sports have increased from an average of 2.1 teams per university in 1972 to 5.6 in 1977 and 7.5 in 1996 ("A Bright Future," 1996). The primary reason for the increase in the number of women sports is that schools had to be in compliance with Title IX. Women's sports should not be earmarked for the consumption of women alone. They have also become attractive to men who are interested in sports.

In general, the demographic future of sport tourism shows signs of booming. The world's population is increasing exponentially, discretionary income is becoming greater in developed countries; a large pool of older adults have money and time on their hands for sports engagement; and women are becoming as much a part of sport tourism as men have been. With cautionary tones included, the signs look good. The demographics are favorable for sport tourism's expansion as long as contributing lifestyle factors help people in their pursuit of sports.

Little has been written about the behaviors and general lifestyle of sport tourists. Therefore, not much can be extrapolated about their future behaviors. With this statement in mind, some tourism trends and consumptive behaviors may provide indicators about future behaviors. In some of these trends, different perspectives and prognosticators offer opposing views. For example, health professionals say that people in developed countries are becoming more sedentary, but the tourism profes-

Motivations, Lifestyles, and Sports Tourism Futures

sionals say that people are demanding more interactive and active tourism opportunities than ever before. People who are active at home will typically seek to be active on vacation.

Motivations versus behavior. Amid the fitness and healthy lifestyle boom in developed countries have been reports of lower levels of fitness and physical activity. Even though many people report regular engagement in exercise, only 37% of so-called "exercisers" do it frequently enough or strenuously enough to gain cardiovascular benefits (Ten Kate, 1995). Some observers say that the increases of quick fixes, such as weight loss remedies, are to blame. Others speculate that increasing dependence on technology creates "couch potatoes." Because of the many sources of sit-down entertainment within homes, people do not have to get off their couches to engage in physical activity. Conversely, when people of developed countries leave their regular environments, they are looking for escape, thrills, risky activities, and challenges.

People involved in motivation research view all the aforementioned desires as the need to escape the regimes of modern life. Escape serves as the antidote to the scheduled, busy, and crowded work world. Thrills, offbeat destinations, and risky activities serve as the antidote to a mundane and routinized existence. As reported by Delpy (1998), participatory or active sport tourists are specifically motivated by escape and relaxation, health and fitness, family togetherness, stress reduction, nature experiences, thrills, and learning. With multiple motivations being evident, the packaging of sport tourism attractions and destinations will need to provide many benefits to accommodate their customers. The locations must be unique and provide activities the sport tourists cannot find at home.

Participating in sport, rather than being a spectator, may be the new trend for the event sport tourists. At some point, spectators will be inclined to try their hand at the game and "just do it." However, packagers of sport tourism must not forget that family tourism is also on the rise. Just like many tourist destinations, variety will be the key for attracting sport tourists. The core sporting activity and attraction will not provide sufficient benefits for people who are trying to escape from their regular lives.

The WTO states that increasingly, tourists are looking for the unique and "non-touristy" places. They also report a dearth of "undiscovered" destinations in the world. The reaction of consumers has been that the highest mountains, the depths of the oceans, the ends of the earth, and outer space are the next big destinations. Mountain-related travel experiences are already possible. Several companies offer tours to destinations with altitude and challenge. The most extreme of these destinations are the countries of Tibet and Nepal where mountain climbing and mountain treks are popular. Even though mountain sports offer great excitement and challenge, commercial operators' taking unprepared "tourists" to the extremes of altitude has caused much debate. As a result of such treks, several accidents have occurred with losses of life being common. Tourists are also plumbing the depths of the ocean. Since 1985, 46 tourist submarines have entered into service, and in 1996, more than 2 million passengers took rides, generating nearly US $147 million in revenues. The current trend in this type of tourism is towards transparent submarines from which patrons can receive better views. The other sporting trend is found in the burgeoning scuba industry. More people are gaining experience in scuba. At the end of the earth is Antarctica, and the WTO predicts this location to be latest extreme destination. In 1997, 10,000 tourists visited the continent, paying between US $ 9,000 and $16,000 for the experience (WTO, 1998a).

Extreme Sports

In 1998, 15 million people watched the ESPN's X Games and many people are now emulating what they saw. There are an estimated 300,000 climbers in the US. In 1988, there was one climbing gym in the US, now there are 400 offering sport climbing. In other sports, freestyle biking has increased in popularity for young males, 9.3 million skateboarders are predicted to be wheeling around America, and there are uncounted thousands of inline skaters. Are these the sports tourists of tomorrow, and the popular sports activities of the future? (McNichol & Soriano, 1998).

Searches for extreme sports are expanding the numbers in skydiving, bungee jumping, and rock climbing. These people tend to be young, above average in income, and single. According to VALS (psychographic research for consumer behavior), these extreme sports people fit into three categories.

1. Full-blooded Experiencers—chase risk for its own sake, adrenaline "junkies"

2. Latent Actualizers—want to experience thrills to challenge themselves

3. Experiencer/Achiever—drawn to extreme sports to win the admiration of others (American Demographics, 1997).

Although escape, thrill, and uniqueness attract some active sport tourists, many event sport tourists are attracted by the pageantry of hallmark sporting events. Variously, these tourists are looking for excellent competition, party environments, cultural differences, and locations with business and historical significance. This type of event is fairly typical of the Olympics, the Superbowl, and the World Cup of Soccer (Delpy, 1998). Although hallmark events surround travelers with sports, pageantry, and people, at a regional level people are also attracted to sports parties contrived by media conglomerates. Partying in a sports atmosphere is what sells out the Baltimore ESPN Zone restaurant every Monday night of football season. People can come to see ABC Monday Night Football being filmed and have the possibility of appearing on television. They also come for the opportunity to see their favorite sports television hosts (Gerstner, 1998).

Luxury vs. value. There appear to be concurrent trends in the consumer travel market with regard to spending. One trend is spending for value, and the other, for luxury. The first is a continuing trend of value-for-money, in which consumers use packaged deals and all-inclusive pricing. By packaging airfares, accommodations, activities, and food, the price becomes more affordable than if they were bought separately. These types of tourism episodes preclude travelers from seeking high-end services, but the price is reduced to a level attainable by middle-income earners. Some of these travelers are seeking luxury, not extreme luxury but enough to make the trip special and different. Coleman (1983) has identified this desire as "sensible snobbery." High-end consumers are not outlandish with their travel purchases but certainly want to be lavished with some sort of luxury while traveling.

The second trend is the demand for high-end, customized tourism services. A small but persistent part of the travel market requires excellence and uniqueness, afforded by spending lots of money. These people are financially well endowed, but they can also be early adopters who are prepared to pay significant proportions of their income to receive the experience first. The trend toward high-end consumption has been caused by a number of events. First, with increasing demands in the workplace and decreasing amounts of time available for travel, tourists are treating themselves to something unique. Second, there is a continuing increase in the discretionary dollars of people from developed countries, and they can spend this on travel and other non-necessities. Third, the reliance on credit is increasing, and the financial impact of consumer tourism spending can be spread over time. The consumers of today are not necessarily extravagant, but they see these escapes as necessities rather than luxuries. In the United States, the rise in consumer spending has continued at a rate of about 4 to 5% per year, with the baby boomers contributing much of the increase. In the near future, the baby boomers will have passed their peak earning years, and they will have more time on their hands for more travel. This phenomenon should fuel the travel market further (Kane, 1999; Oldenburg, 1999).

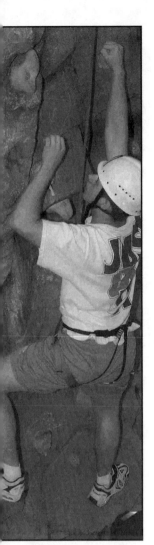

Climbing walls have become common in gyms throughout the U.S.

Photo reprinted by permission of John Bright Images.

Time crunch. Although several studies have reported that people have less leisure time than ever before (e.g., Schor, 1991), a recent study (Godbey & Robinson, 1998) suggests that people have about the same amount of leisure time. Today, however, that time is so fragmented that it decreases the opportunity for meaningful and extended leisure. Therefore, shorter, more frequent vacations and weekend travel will continue to increase as people have difficulty scheduling long vacations together. The time crunch is exacerbated by two-career families, children's school schedules, asynchronous vacations between partners, and different hours of work (Schor). Sport planners who schedule events over weekends may be able to entice other family members along with those who participate in the sports. The WTO reports that with less leisure time but more discretionary money available, tourists will be searching for "high thrills quickly." This problem of less leisure time is particularly noticeable in the United States (see Table 6). In European countries, paid vacations are considerably longer. Nevertheless, the WTO has identified diminishing leisure time as a trend of the future.

Table 10.5. Average Number of Vacation Days of Countries Around the World

Italy	42 Days
France	37 Days
Germany	35 Days
Brazil	34 Days
United Kingdom	28 Days
Canada	26 Days
Korea	25 Days
Japan	25 Days
USA	13 Days

Source: Travel Industry of America

In the future, people are going to be money rich but time poor (WTO Business Council, 1998). After studying 18 countries that represent 73% of the world's spending, the WTO found that people are working longer hours because companies are facing more global competition. According to Jose Luis Zoreda, chief executive of the World Tourism Organization Business Council, "the effect of this squeeze on leisure time will be to accelerate the trend to shorter, more frequent holidays. It will also favor the expansion of quickly accessible holiday destinations in the same time region or time zone." Leisure time constraints for the prospective tourist works against most distant (long-haul) destinations vying for the sport tourism market. Although vacation time is not necessarily indicative of all free time, it provides sufficient blocks where people can travel for sports.

Geographics/Environment

One of the biggest sport tourism threats comes from the degradation of the environment. According to Weiner (1990), a five-degree change in temperature will directly affect lives of the people all over the world. Evidence of ozone loss is already affecting the outdoor activities of Australians and New Zealanders. Burn times for direct exposure to the sun have been reduced dramatically, and skin cancer is a real concern.

At the 1998 WTO World Congress on Snow and Winter Sports Tourism, the key concern was the effect of global warming on the ski industry. It was said that climatic change caused by global warming would affect lower altitude ski resorts with an estimated loss of US$2 billion to a country such as Switzerland. With warming temperatures, snow cover will recede to higher elevations and will last for fewer months of the year. This could be very costly to a market that has 15–20 million international travelers and four times that number of domestic visitors (WTO, 1998b).

Within the next 30 to 50 years, available skiing areas will become crowded. However, it is also expected that ski areas will not lose their revenues through shortened seasons. Technological enhancements to generate snow and chemical enhancements to replace snow are likely to be developed, as are new ski technologies to take advantage of these changes. Also expected are tourism movements towards northern and southern extremes for real snow. Concerns over the negative environmental impacts of ski area (e.g., deforestation, pollution), and golf course developments (disruption of wildlife habitat, ground and surface water contamination from pesticides and herbicides) have forced governmental jurisdictions to require careful study and planning for future projects.

The depletion of the world's ozone layer is projected by many to cause changes other than loss of snow cover. The water of the world will rise and engulf many of the traditional areas that are used for water sports. In the United States, a large portion of the Mississippi River valley will also be under water. Cities on the coasts of most countries will be severely affected., and people will need to move to higher elevations, a migration that will create additional crowding on available land. Areas closer to the equator may become parched. Climate changes in other areas will alter vegetation. Storms and climatic disturbances will also change the nature of many outdoor sports.

Although the changes in climate will have a devastating impact on sport tourism, reductions of animal species will also have negative consequences for sport. One third of all animal species have become extinct during the past 100 years. Game fish and land animals will need to change their migration patterns or habitats to adjust. Sport fishing and hunting have to adjust or die out due to the changed habitats of the animals.

| **Technology and Sport Tourism Futures** | The World Tourism Organization's chief of statistics, Enzo Paci expects that tourism will become the antidote for high tech living in the next century. With technology invading every aspect of our lives, we become increasingly cut off from other people because machines can provide us with most of what we need. What machines cannot provide is the basic |

need for human interaction and Paci believes that tourism will be a conduit for this to happen. In the same statement, Paci speculates that technology will assist people with their travel. He predicts that "short pleasure voyages to outer space will become a reality by 2004 or 2005." A four day trip will cost about US $100,000 and some companies are already taking reservations and deposits. Even so, Paci further states that only 7% of the world's population will be traveling internationally by 2020, which is double that of 1996.

Technology is one of the least predictable areas for the discussion on the future of sport tourism. Innovations are happening so rapidly that it is difficult to predict technological changes in the future. We would do well to remind ourselves about the words of an early International Business Machines (IBM) president. His statement was that computers would not be a viable commercial entity until they could be made to weigh under $1^1/_2$ tons.

With caveats in place, there are four areas where technological development will create major changes in sport tourism. The effects of the first three are difficult to project, but the fourth is already upon us. The first three areas are the reaction to and the development of sustainable energy; the reaction to and the development of biogenetic engineering; and the development of transportation that is faster, larger, and more economic. The fourth and final technological development is information technology. Satellites, the Internet, and computers are already changing the way information is distributed, received, and collected.

Fossil fuels are projected for exhaustion in the 21st century and have also been the cause of global pollution. In lieu of fossil fuels, new forms of sustainable energy are being developed. Some of these forms are the separation of water into its component parts, solar energy through the sun's radiation, and wind energy. But what types of sport tourism will be affected by the demise of fossil fuel? By definition, sport tourism implies travel, and therefore, all sports will be affected even if fossil fuels are not related to the activity. Combustible power sources will need to find new energy sources other than oil and natural gas. This will affect various forms of transportation (also racing) in the air, on the ground, and in the water. Although technology will likely find ways to create power from other sources, speeds and duration of travel will be inhibited in the short term. These constraints will not be technological as much as they will be related to affordability. Given the concern about fossil fuels, travelers using them will be taxed or limited in their use. On the positive side, new fuels may create new sports related to the use of the sun and the wind.

Source: www.world-tourism.org/newslett/nov97/vis2020.htm

An ethical dilemma in sports will be created by the technological marvels of cloning, biogenetic engineering, and chemical engineering. Already, sports people are using undetectable chemicals to enhance performance. It is merely a matter of time before biogenetic engineering produces superhuman athletes. If sports become the domain of super humans, will spectators feel disconnected? Will the average person identify with the athletes and travel to see them compete?

Of the non-information technology futures, the impacts of transportation are the closest at hand. Sport tourists will be able to travel farther, faster, cheaper, and in greater volume than ever before. Supersonic, ozone altitude planes will transport individuals in great numbers to distances further afield and in shorter periods of time. The ease of transportation will allow spectators and participants to engage in nonnative sports as easily as sports in their own areas. Major sports will move beyond the realm of being regionalized by their continents and will become globalized. Professional leagues have already spread over the continents with teams from the Super Twelve Rugby competition being located in South Africa, Australia, and New Zealand.

The greatest advances are happening in information technology. Not only is information doubling in volume every five years, but it is also becoming more accessible. One can expound upon the development of the Internet as a prime mover in this field, but the reality is that all forms of information technology are advancing. With news and information accessible all over the world, sporting activities will be available to everyone. Information access will allow the sport tourist to follow games on other continents, have sporting heroes who are thousands of miles away, and follow sports that were once the domain of their own region only. Access to sports information may increase interest in seeing live competitions. On the other hand, if information technology becomes so good that a viewer can see and feel the excitement of the game, many events may become staged without the presence of spectators.

Although advanced technology may be a threat to sport tourism, consumers seem to seek "high touch" as the world becomes more "high tech." Whatever the outcome, information technology will allow individuals with lower incomes to follow their favorite events. Information technology will also break the barriers of differences in language. It is expected that technology will be used to translate electronically any sports broadcast into the language of the consumer, thereby negating the need for many sports announcers.

Advances in virtual reality may also cause a boom or a bust for sport tourism. The notion of "try before you buy" may negate the need to visit sporting events. On the other hand, virtual reality may increase the demand for seeing a real event and more human contact. Live sports may well become a "snob good" where enthusiasts want to "keep up with the Joneses."

Information technology advances are already having an effect on the traditional providers of tourism. Travel agents are in decline as consumers reserve their travel plans on the Internet. Already available on the Internet are reservations for tee times (Wright, 1998), airlines, tickets, rental cars, and accommodations. Furthermore, reservations will be made during a person's free time instead of during business time.

Projections for Internet shopping are increasing rapidly. Experts say that Internet shopping will reflect traditional shopping but not to the demise of traditional shops. Some items will still need to be tried in person before being bought. In 1997, US $5 billion was spent on the Internet with an estimated US $95.1 billion by 2002. The potential for growth is tremendous. By 2002, 22% of US households will use Internet services, but only 30% of those will make purchases on the Internet. Travel has been the biggest winner for Internet business thus far. Consumers can compare fares to get the best deals, and tourism is not something that can be tried out in a store before being sold. By buying through the Internet

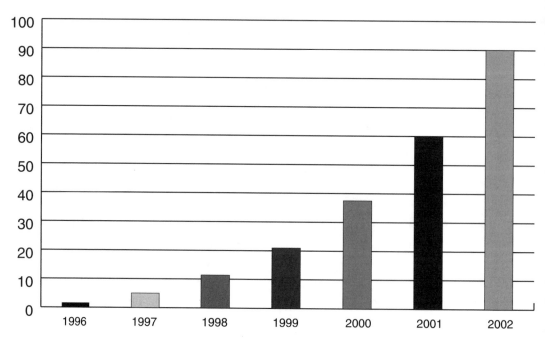

Figure 10.4. International Spending on the Internet (billions)

Table 10.6. Projected Growth of Travel Revenue on the Internet (US$ billions)

Year	Revenue
1996	0.3
1997	0.8
1998	1.9
1999	3.2
2000	4.7
2001	6.5
2002	8.9

rather than relying on an agent who works on commission, consumers can obtain special deals and know what they are getting. (Lourosa, 1998).

Actual Internet spending in 1997 was $997 million, which tripled sales from the previous year. The potential for online travel is still enormous, as the money spent was only 1% of all travel expenditures. Eighty-four percent of all online sales were airline tickets (Travel Industry Association of America [TIA], 1998). In 1998, 70 million Americans used the Internet for travel purposes, which was a 184% increase in 2 years. Ninety-two percent of those Internet users took trips of 100+ miles that year (TIA, 1998). With the most prolific group of Internet users being youth and children, they will be next great consumer group in the world, travel included.

Sport Tourism Marketing

Fifty percent of sport tourists attend a professional event, and the other 50% travel to attend amateur events (Delpy, 1998). Not only do marketers need to be active in professional sports, but they must also be active in the amateur disciplines. As sport tourism dollars become recognized for

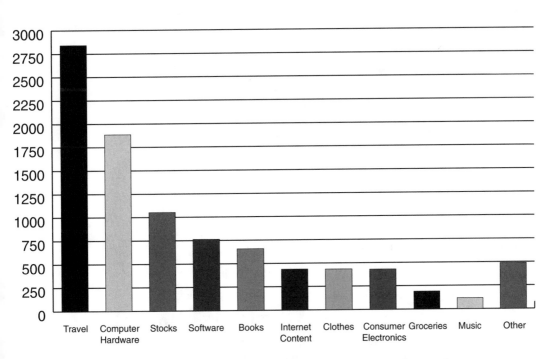

Figure 10.5. Unitered States Internet Spending Comparisons by Products—1998 (millions)

their economic impacts, and growth, competition will become keen amongst marketers. They will have to know more about the populations they are trying to attract, and they will also have to entice additional markets who are not core customers.

Marketing is often misunderstood. For many people, marketing is synonymous with advertising and promotion, whereas those activities are usually towards the end of the marketing process. Marketing is the process of planning and implementing a product or service to be sold. It also entails determining what consumers want and the price that people can afford to pay, and developing sufficient revenue to meet organizational goals. Other activities include promoting the product or service and finding a way to most efficiently and effectively distribute it to consumers to maximize their satisfaction. Finally, it is following up with consumers to find out if they are satisfied with their purchase. To this end, organizations need to find out who wants their products or services, what they want, and where those products or services can be most conveniently delivered.

The growth of the sport tourism phenomenon has led to a growth in the sophistication of its marketing and delivery. It has also led to a growth of those sports wishing to profit from the potential tourism dollars that are available. With many sports entering the sport tourism arena, the market will become saturated with options, and marketers will have to differentiate their events to attract visitors. Overabundance in the sport tourism market is not critical yet because there are many untapped tourists out there. However, attracting mass audiences with mass marketing will become increasingly difficult. Consider this incomplete list of sports played in the United States that are already professional and have a market presence within the marketplace:

American Football	Automobile Racing	Baseball
Basketball	Cycling—road	Dance
Dog and Horse Racing	Fishing	Golf
Gymnastics	Ice Hockey	Ice Skating
Lacrosse	Martial Arts	Motorcycle Racing
Mountain Biking	Pool or Billiards	In-line Skating
Sailing	Skateboarding	Skiing (downhill)
Soccer	Softball Snowboarding	Surfing
Tennis	10-pin Bowling	Track and Field
Volleyball		

The array of sports trying to attract tourists may need to widen their catchment area to include nonsports fans. These consumers will come to the games for the spectacle, entertainment, or social reasons, and not just for the contests. Unfortunately, increased "entertainment" may alienate sports fanatics as the core attraction becomes increasingly muddied by peripheral entertainment. The marketing sophistication of professional and major sports may also divert attention from many minor and amateur sports that have held previously prominent positions. In the United States, track and field events have lost much of their market share to other sports.

It is not clear the extent to which one form of sport tourism (active, event-based, celebratory) contributes to (or detracts from) the popularity of another form of sport tourism. For example, to what extent does a golf vacation lead to PGA tournament attendance, or being a die-hard Chicago Cubs leads to visiting the Major League Baseball Hall of Fame? It is surmised that there is a symbiotic relationship across the three forms of sport tourism, though future research should investigate the direction of sport tourist behaviors across these areas.

An alternative for less prominent sports is to use marketing strategies that focus on locations of intermediate size where they are not competing against sports with a strong market presence. This has been very successful for minor league baseball and basketball teams. Another alternative is to play the sports in a nontraditional season so there is less competition with prominent sports. It is here that the notion of developing nontraditional consumers and niche marketing arises. According to Getz (1998), niche marketing is based on attracting narrow groups of potential sports consumers. Nontraditional sports consumers may be a group that has not been considered previously. In the next paragraph are some examples that illustrate attempts to attract nontraditional or niche markets.

Minor league baseball has always been located in smaller cities where there is little competition from other sports. In recent years, however, the emphasis has changed from baseball fans to events tailored for the entire family. The marketing thrust is the developing of a package that will attract entire families for inexpensive evenings of sport, not too far from home. Another sport that is attempting to attract nontraditional consumers is skiing. The previous boom in skiing is diminishing as baby boomers retire, become less active, and move to other activities. The ski industry is not only trying to attract a new group of young skiers through snowboarding, but they are also trying to attract ethnic groups who have not previously skied in large numbers. For example, the goal for the Vail, Colorado, is to increase the participation of minorities to

10% of the US ski market within 5 years. Because U.S. minorities account for $1 trillion in disposable income, the ski industry has planned promotional efforts in Miami (second largest packaged ski market), Dallas, Chicago, and Los Angeles, especially to young minorities (Blum, 1998). Even major professional sports are trying to attract an ethnically diverse set of consumers as the demographics of the population changes. Many professional sports appear to be signing athletes who mirror the ethnic background of their population catchment area (Lombardo, 1998).

Another niche market will be the older adults and retired athletes who have plenty of time on their hands and plenty of discretionary income to spend. Although their ability to participate has diminished, the will to participate has not. Therefore, the nostalgia sports market will become increasingly popular with those who want to maintain contact with their sport (Getz, 1998).

The Rise of the NASCAR Fan Base

Perhaps the largest market barriers to increased sport tourism are related to competition from other free-time activities. In addition, Delpy (1998) has reported several personal barriers to sport tourism and sport participation. Those barriers are lacks of time, interest, money, ticket availability, and accommodations; cost; and distance.

Robinson (1998) claimed that the arts are competing for spectators more than ever before. If this trend continues, traditional sports locations may consider it cheaper to build a performing arts center or an art gallery than a sports stadium. Once considered the domain of the upper classes, arts are becoming more widespread among various populations, and attendance at cultural events is on the increase. Other activities may also impinge upon the traditional consumer segments of sport tourism, especially if they alleviate some of the personal barriers that sport tourists encounter when trying to participate.

Additional competition will also intensify between communities seeking to attract and retain sport championships and the sport tourists. The high demand for hosting large-scale sporting events has created a "seller's market" for the International Olympic Committee, professional leagues, amateur sporting associations, and other governing bodies. For example, 30 cities bid to host the 1998 U.S. Weightlifting Association's Olympic Trials. For more high-profile sporting events, including the NCAA Final Four Men's Basketball Championships and the U.S. Summer Olympic Track and Field Trials, communities interested in hosting the events must provide large dollar amounts as "up-front" guarantees. Communities interested in hosting sporting events have established sport commissions to present a unified front for their formal bid proposals. Whether youth sporting events will command similar financial commitments is uncertain. Market forces will determine whether youth sports are priced too high or are highly desirable.

The personal barriers are issues that sport marketers need to deal with more effectively when promoting their events. Ever since services marketing became differentiated from product marketing, these issues have been paramount concerns. Lack of time and money, and too much distance are barriers linked to sport tourism delivery. In services marketing, there have been three traditional solutions:

1. Move the service closer to the consumer;

2. Have the service connected to the consumer through an intermediary such as electronic communication; or

3. Bring the consumer to the service.

Unfortunately, none of options helps sport tourism as they all eliminate the need for travel. These options can be used to help with travel preparation and planning, but they negate the need for travel if they become ubiquitous. Some visionaries say that this is already happening through television and the Internet. The challenge for sport tourism marketers will be to transport sport tourists to the event quickly, conveniently, and inexpensively. This is a large challenge. Anyone who has tried to travel great distances already knows that airline schedules and flight plans are not always convenient.

Lack of ticket availability and accommodations is another major constraint especially for mega or hallmark sporting events. Unfortunately, sports venues and the associated accommodations are capacity constrained, allowing only a certain number of people to participate as spectators or participants. Accommodations can hold only a certain number of people as can sport venues. The obvious answer has been the electronic communication of the event to interested people, but this again negates the need for travel. Building more hotels and larger stadiums is probably not feasible because the venues would need to be used very frequently to make them economically viable. Such is the problem for sport tourism marketers. How do they eliminate barriers so that people can travel easily, and how do they deal with the demand when they have successfully promote the event?

Sport Tourism Marketplace

Sport tourism marketing and the sport tourism marketplace are very different even though the names sound the same. The sport tourism marketplace refers to what is to be sold in terms of services and products. It not only refers to the sporting events but also to the venues and the organizations involved. This section covers potential future of sporting event types, the future of sport locations and venues, and the changes in the organizations involved in sport tourism.

Although some sports will change locations because of global warming or the desire to become closer to their base of consumers, other sports will change locations to take advantage of different surroundings. The most advanced of the predictions to date discusses the notion of sports in space ("Space Future," 1998). Imagine the changes that will take place because of weightlessness and the need for carrying oxygen. If one thinks about traditional sports being played in space, arenas will have to be expanded two- or threefold, because weightless athletic feats will carry people, footballs, and golf balls much farther than earthbound efforts do. Rules and refereeing will need complete overhauls to handle the lack of gravity and oxygen. Perhaps rulebooks will have to be rewritten with records that denote gravitational and nongravitational feats. More likely, however, is the development of totally different sporting activities that take advantage of the unique properties of space. For sport tourism, the most likely early scenario relates to people traveling into space to experience sporting feats they could not manage at home. The early sport tourist will be confined to those who can afford to pay large sums of money to travel skyward. At this time, sport participation in space is more foreseeable than is the mass transit of spectators into space. Perhaps this is the next frontier of extreme sports and the media-generated X Games.

In the near future and already evident in some places, sports "Meccas" will become popular. Just as Disney World has made Orlando, Florida, the mecca of contrived tourism experiences, it is also becoming a mecca of sports entertainment. Sports meccas will partially solve the spectator space and accommodation constraints experienced by other locations because they can fill many hotels rooms and venues with other types of tourists too. As a result, they will also create sports ghost towns in geographically close locations that are trying to compete (Maguire, 1998). The advantage for individual sport tourists and for groups will be that they can experience many different sports in one location. There will be a sporting activity to suit everyone. The other advantage is that high-volume travel to a few destinations will make travel more direct and less expensive. Already, airfares to Orlando, Florida, are cheap by comparison with those to other places.

The reaction to the threat of sport tourism meccas is occurring already as cities, local governments, and professional franchises establish partnerships to compete. They, collectively, are trying to obtain parts of the projected economic boom that comes with visitors to sporting events (Pickard, 1999). In a world already competing heavily for the rights to host sporting events (think of the efforts that have been expended to capture the Olympics, legally or otherwise), partnerships will be necessary to build facilities, generate the large promotion necessary, and finance the event. (Getz, 1998; Mullen, 1998). Federal governments are "buying into" these partnerships to stimulate local and regional economic growth through sport tourism. The Canadian Sport Tourism Initiative is building partnerships in communities to garner the economic benefits of sport. The Canadian Sport Tourism Initiative is primarily interested in attracting international sports because the communities can make more money by creating add-on packages that extend visitors' stays. This creates additional economic benefits, gives communities worldwide exposure, and enhances the local quality of life through local improvement and facility building (Canadian Tourism Commission, 1997).

As federal governments are accepting the premise that sport tourism is good for local economies, so are the cities. Sometimes cities have been forced to support sports and sport tourism. In order to maintain these benefits, some sporting bodies have held cities at ransom with regard to building new facilities. If the facilities are not built, the team or the sport leaves town, and the benefits are lost. The financial commitment can be much higher than the cost of a brand-new facility. Good roads, improved airports, parking lots, and accommodations are all part of the package to be competitive in the face of increasing competition. These improvements are being financed in large part by cities and their taxpayers. Although this trend is already occurring in professional sports, amateur sports with potential for drawing large groups will likely leverage similar clout in the future.

In return for excellent facilities and city support, it is likely that these venues will encourage peripheral commercial opportunities that will extend the financial season of the sport and the community. Extended seasons can be developed by

1. Locating team personnel, headquarters, practice and/or preseason training facilities in the community so that people travel to see their team in periods beyond the season;

2. Creating facilities that will be multipurpose or at least dual purpose with the ability to host other types of events (e.g., Super Bowl, NCAA Men's Basketball Final Four, NBA All-Star Game); and

3. Extending the financial season through vertical integration of accommodations, hospitality, and related retail businesses (Turco & Ostrosky, 1997).

Another trend, especially in the professional ranks of sport, is media and communications empires' becoming the owners of teams. Although sponsorship and advertising were once the preferred representation of these empires, corporations see many benefits in ownership. Corporations' buying professional teams is good for their media businesses. Through ownership or majority investment, media empires will have exclusive control over the broadcast rights. This is already happening with in a number of cases:

• Rupert Murdoch's empire owns the Los Angeles Dodgers, is the corporate backer of Super Twelve rugby, and has previously bid on the Manchester United soccer team.

• The Disney Corporation owns professionals teams as does the Turner Group.

• An American company, NTL Cable has bid $269 million for the Newcastle United soccer team, and WGN Broadcasting also owns professional sporting franchises (Kaplan, 1998).

The result of greater media influence will likely change the nature of sports to make it more palatable for global audiences. It is also predicted that professional sports will consider the spectators as second in priority to television, video, and the Internet, because the revenues these sources generate will dwarf spectator admissions (Dortch, 1996).

The future influences on sport tourism are too numerous to mention and very uncertain. Even though demographics, the environment, technology, and marketing have been mentioned in this chapter, it is hard to envision how they will change the overall sport tourism environment. Presented in this chapter were a few scenarios, but many others have not even been conceived at this writing. Perhaps the greatest uncertainty of all is politics. Although not mentioned in this chapter, will the politics of commercialism, nationalism, and ethnic difference be a driving force for the expansion of sport tourism, or will it lead to unhealthy division and conflict? Whatever the face of sport tourism in the future, it will be more commercialized, more accessible, and more pervasive in the modern world.

References

A bright future for women in sports: Forecast. (1996, September). American Demographics [Online]. Available: www.demographics.com/publications/fc/96_fc/9609_fc/9609f02.htm

A call for leadership. (1988, August 17). *VeloNews* [Online]. Available: www.velonews.com [1998, September 5].

Advertisement for themed sports cruises. (1998, June 25). *Travel Weekly, 57*(53). p. 17.

Alesch, D. J. (1995*). The Green Bay Packers: America's only not-for-profit, major league sports franchise*. Milwaukee: The Wisconsin Policy Research Institute.

Anything Packers creates record $130 million in sales. (1997, April 4*). Green Bay Press-Gazette*, p. A-2.

Arnold, M. (Winter 1995). The state of admission criteria to doctoral granting institutions in the field of recreation, park, and leisure studies. *Society of Park and Recreation Educators Newsletter, 1995.* p. 4.

Arnold, M., & Bartlett, K. (October, 1996*). From gown to town: Making the transition from college to workforce*. Presentation at the National Park and Recreation Association Conference, Kansas City.

Assael, H. (1987). *Consumer behavior and marketing action*. Boston, MA: PWS Kent.

Baade, R. A. (1996). Professional sports as catalysts for metropolitan economic development. *Journal of Urban Affairs, 18*(1), 1–16.

Baade, R. A. (1994). *Stadiums, professional sports, and economic development: Assessing reality*. Detroit: The Heartland Institute.

Backstrom, C. H., & Hursh-Cesar, G. (1981). *Survey research*. New York: John Wiley & Sons.

Ball says IOC has repaid Athens debt by granting it 2004 Games (1997, September 8). *Pretoria News,* p. 3.

Berlonghi, A. (1990). *The special event risk management manual.* Dana Point, CA: Berlonghi.

Berry, L., & Parasuraman, A. (1991). *Marketing services: Competing through quality*. New York: Free Press.

Bitner, M., Booms, J., & Tetreault, B. (1990). The service encounter: Diagnosing favorable and unfavorable incidents. *Journal of Marketing, 54*, 71–84.

Blalock, H. M., & Wilken, P. H. (1979). *Intergroup processes: A micro-macro perspective*. New York: Free Press.

Blum, E. (1998, July 13). Vail resorts steps up efforts to attract minorities to the slopes. Travel Weekly, 57(55), 10.

Bridges, F. J., & Roquemore, L. L. (1992). *Management for athletic/sport administration*. Decatur, GA: ESM.

Brooks, C. (1994). Sports marketing: Competitive business strategies for sports. Englewood Cliffs, NJ: Prentice Hall.

Brown, J. (1998, March 15). More lines catch on to allure of golf sailing. *Travel Weekly, 57*(15), c3.

Brundtland, K.R. (1988). Getting value from plan reviews. In *Getting value from strategic planning* [Research Report No. 915]. New York: The Conference Board. P. 163–179.

Burns, J. P. A., & Mules, T. J. (1989). An economic evaluation of the Adelaide Grand Prix. In G. J. Syme, B. J. Shaw, P. M. Fenton, & W. S. Mueller (Eds.), *The planning and evaluation of hallmark events* (pp. 172–185). Aldershort, England: Avebury.

Cameron, J (1998). Tourism highlights/Points salliant touristiques 7–13 Nov. 1998. Cameron.Judith@ic.gc.ca posted to TRINET-L@hawaii.edu.

Canadian Tourism Commission (1997). Sports tourism to tap into billion dollar market [Online]. Available: _ HYPERLINK 206.191.33.50/tourism/news/17jn97.html 206.191.33.50/tourism/news/17jn97.html_

Catherwood, D.W., & Van Kirk, R.L. (1992). *The complete guide to special event management.* New York: John Wiley and Sons.

Cato, B. & Crotts, J. (1993). Experimenting with discount pricing. *Parks and Recreation, 27*(12), 30–34, 67.

Citrine, K. (1995). Site planning for events. In *Event operations* (pp. 17–19). Port Angeles, WA: International Festivals and Events Association.

Coakley. J. (1998). *Sports in society: Issues and controversies* (6th ed.). Boston, MA: Irwin McGraw Hill.

Cobb, S. & Weinberg, D. (1993). The importance of import substitution in regional economic impact analysis: Empirical estimates from two Cincinnati area events. *Economic Development Quarterly, 7*(3), 282–6.

Coleman, R. (1983). The continuing significance of social class to marketing. *Journal of Consumer Research, 10,* 265–280.

Cook, D., Melcher, R. A., & Welling, B. (1987, August 31). Nothing sells like sports: Business pours billions into fun and games. *Business Week,* 48–53.

Cooper, C., et al. 1994. The Destination Life Cycle: An Update. In *Tourism: The State of the Art.* A. V. Seaton, ed. Pp. 342–346. Chichester, England: Wiley.

Copeland, R. P. (1991). Sport sponsorship in Canada: A study of exchange between corporate sponsors and sport groups. Unpublished master's thesis, University of Waterloo, Waterloo, Ontario, Canada.

Crompton, J. (1979). Motivations for pleasure vacation. *Annals of Tourism Research, 7*(4), 408–424.

Crompton, J. L. (1981, March). How to find the price that's right. *Parks and Recreation,* 32–39, 64.

Crompton, J. L. (1984). Voluntary retrenchment of park and recreation services. *Journal of Park and Recreation Administration, 2*(3), 10–20.

Crompton, J. L. (1995). Economic impact analysis of sport facilities and events: Eleven sources of misapplication. *Journal of Sport Management, 9,* 14–35.

Crompton, J. L., & Ap, J. (1994). *Development of a tourism impact scale in host resident context* [Research Enhancement Program Final Report]. College Station, TX: Texas A&M University.

Crompton, J. L., & Lamb, C. W. (1986). *Marketing government and social services.* New York: John Wiley & Sons.

Crothers, T. (1995, June 19). The shakedown: Greedy owners threatening to move their teams. *Sports Illustrated,* 8–80.

Cunningham, M. H., & Taylor, S. F. (1995). Event marketing: State of the industry and research agenda. *Festival Management and Event Tourism, 2*(3/4), 123–137.

Davis, J. (1996). NASCAR—Winston Cup [Online]. Available: :cnnfn.com/hotstories/bizbuz/9611/18/nascar_pkg/index.htm

Davis, K.A. (1994). *Sport management: Successful private sector business strategies*. Dubuque, IA: W.C. Brown.

De Knopf, P., & Standevan, J. (1998). *Sport tourism*. Champaign, IL: Human Kinetics.

Delpy, L. (1997, June). *Winning the game: The rise of sports tourism*. Paper presented at the 28th Annual Travel and Tourism Research Association Conference, Norfolk, VA.

Delpy, L. (1998, August 17–23). Sport tourism. *Street and Smith's Sport Business* 17(1), 31–34.

Disney complex beckons sports fans. (1997, November 13). *Travel Weekly, 56*(90), pT8.

Dortch, S. (1996). The future of baseball. American Demographics [Online]. Available: www.demographics.com/publications/ad96_ad/9604_ad/9604af01.htm

Doxey, G. (1975) A causation theory of visitor-residents irritants: methodology and research inferences. *The Impact of Tourism, Sixth Annual Conference Proceedings of the Travel Research Association*. San Diego, pp. 195–198.

Ensor, R. J. (1987, September). The corporate view of sports sponsorship. *Athletic Business*, 40–43.

Farmer, P.J., Mulrooney, A.L., & Ammon, Jr., R. (1996). *Sport facility planning and management*. Morgantown, WV: Fitness Information Technologies.

Farr, J., Ludden, L., & Mangin, P. (1997). *The enhanced occupational outlook handbook*. Indianapolis, IN: JIST Works, Inc.

Fleck, S. (1996). Events without barriers: Customer service is a key in complying with the American with Disabilities Act. In *Festivals* (pp. 34–35). Port Angeles, WA: International Festivals and Events Association.

Fox, J. (1996, May). Safety in sports grounds. *The safety & health practitioner*, 26–29.

Friedman, A. (1990, December). Sport marketers must work harder and smarter to score. *Athletic Business*, p. 22.

Gammon, S. & Robinson, T. (1997). Sports and tourism: A conceptual framework. *Journal of Sports Tourism, 4*(3), 8–15. Available online: www.freepress.com/journals/jst/vol4no3

Gazel, R. C. & Schwer, R. K. (1997). Beyond rock and roll: The economic impact of the Grateful Dead on a local economy. *Journal of Cultural Economics, 21*, 41–55.

Gerstner, J. (1998, Nov. 23). ESPNZone gives fans prime view. USA Today, p. 3C

Getz, D. (1997). *Event management and event tourism*. New York: Cognizant Communication Corporation.

Getz, D. (1998). Trends, strategies, and issues in sport-event tourism. *Sport Marketing Quarterly*, 7(2),10–13.

Gibson, H. (1998a). Active sport tourism: Who participates? *Leisure Studies, 17*, 2, 155–170.

Gibson, H. (1998b). Sport tourism: A critical analysis of research. *Sport Management Review, 1*, 45–76.

Gibson, H., Attle, S. & Yiannakis, A. (1998). Segmenting the sport tourist market: A life span perspective. *Journal of Vacation Marketing, 4*, 52–64.

Goldblatt, J. J. (1997). *Special events best practices in modern event management*. New York: Van Nostrand Reinhold.

Government of South Africa, Department of Environmental Affairs and Tourism (1996). *White Paper: Development and Promotion of Tourism in South Africa*. Pretoria: RSA.

Glyptis, S. A. (1991). "Sport and Tourism." In Progress in Tourism, Recreation and Hospitality Management, Volume Three, edited by C. P. Cooper. London: Belhaven Press, pp. 165–83.

Graham, S., Goldblatt, J. J., & Delpy, L. (1995). *The ultimate guide to sport event management & marketing*. New York: Irwin Professional Publishing.

Gunn, C. (1988). *Tourism planning.* New York: Taylor Francis.

Hall, C. M. (1989). Hallmark events and the planning process. In G. J. Syme, B. J. Shaw, D. M. Fenton, & W. S. Mueller, W. S. (Eds.), *The planning and evaluation of hallmark events* (pp. 20–39). Aldershot: Avesbury

Hall, C. M. (1992). *Hallmark tourist events, impacts, management and planning.* London: Bellhaven.

Howard, D. R. & Crompton, J. L. (1995). *Financing sport.* Morgantown, WV: Fitness Information Technology, Inc.

Hudman, L. E. & Hawkins, D. E. (1989). *Tourism in Contemporary Society.* Englewood Cliffs, New Jersey: Prentice-Hall.

International Events Group. (2001). Sponsorship update. [Available online: www.sponsorship.com].

International Events Group. (1996). *IEG Sponsorshop Report, 14*(24), 1–2.

International Events Group. (1997). *IEG's complete guide to sponsorship.* Chicago: IEG, Inc.

International Olympic Committee (2000). *Manual for Cities Bidding for the Olympic Games.* Lucerne: IOC.

Irwin, R. L. and Asimakopoulos, M. K. (1992) "An Approach to the Evaluation and Selection of Sport Sponsorship Proposals", *Sport Marketing Quarterly*, Vol. 1 No. 2, pp. 43–51.

Irwin, R. L. & Sutton, W. A. (1994). Sport sponsorship objectives: An analysis of their relative importance for major corporate sponsors. *European Journal for Sport Management, 1*(2), 93–101.

Iso Ahola, S. (1984). *Leisure counseling: Implications and applications.* Springfield, IL: Charles C. Thomas.

Johnson, R. (1992). How the Chicago Mayor's Office of Special Events uses surveys in its sponsorship program. *IEG Sponsorship Report, 11*(1), 4–5.

Kane, M. (1999, March 28). Inconspicuous consumption characterizes new consumer. *Syracuse Herald American*, pp. E1, E8.

Kaplan, D. (1998, Sept. 21–27). Price tag for Yankees could reach $1 billion. *Street and Smith's Sports Business Journal, 1*(22), 1,43.

Kraus, R. (1997). *Recreation and leisure in modern society*, Sudbury, MA: Jones & Bartlett Publishers.

Kraus, R. & Curtis, J. *Creative management in recreation, parks, and leisure services.* St. Louis: McGraw-Hill.

Korean National Tourist Office. www.knto.or.kr/0knto/future.htm

Kurtzman, J. & Zauhar, J. (1997). A wave in time: The sports tourism phenomena. *Journal of Sports Tourism, 4*(2), 5–20. Available online: mcb.co.uk/journals/jst/archive/vol4no2/welcome.htm#BS4

Kurtzman, J. (1997). Sport tourism consumer motivation. *Journal of Sports Tourism, 4*(3), 13–24. Available online: free-press.com/journals/jst/vol4no3/jst15.htm#BS6

Kuzma, J. R., Shanklin, W. L. & McCally, J. F. (1993). Number one principle for sporting events seeking corporate sponsors: Meet benefactor's objectives. *Sport Marketing Quarterly, 2*(3), 27–37.

Lane, R. (1994, June). Bread and circuses. *Forbes, 153,* 62–64.

Letscher, M (1997). Sports fads and trends. www_.demographics.com/publications/ad/97_ad/9706_ad/ad/970632.htm

Levine, J. (1988). Sports sponsorships: Maximizing the potential. *Incentive, 162,* 6, 30–37.

Lombardo, J. (1998). Courting a different crowd. *Street and Smiths Sports Business*, 1(2) pp. 19–20, May 4–10.

Lourosa, C. (1998). Change in store. *Wall Street Journal*, November, 16, p. R28.

Lovelock, C. (1984). *Services marketing.* Englewood Cliffs, NJ: Prentice Hall.

Madden, P., & Grube, J. (1994). The frequency and nature of alcohol and tobacco advertising in televised sports, 1990 through 1992. *American Journal of Public Health, 84*(2), 297–299.

Maguire, C. (1998). Disney's sport mecca puts other cities on the defense. *Street and Smith's Sport Business Journal*, September 21–27, 1(22), p. 8

Matras, J. (1973). Population and societies. Englewood Cliffs, NJ: Prentice Hall

Mayfield, T. L., & Crompton, J. L. (1995). Development of an instrument for identifying community reasons for staging a festival. *Journal of Travel Research, 34*(1), 37–44.

McCarville, R. E. (1993). Successful pricing is in the eye of the beholder. *Parks and Recreation, 27*(12), 36–40.

McCarville, R. E., & Copeland, R. P. (1994). Understanding sport sponsorship through exchange theory. *Journal of Sport Management*, 8, 102–114.

McNichol, T., & Soriano, C. (1998). USA Weekend, July 24–26, p. 14.

McCook, K., Turco, D., & Riley, R. (1997). Corporate decision making processes involving sport sponsorship proposals. *Cyber-Journal of Sport Marketing, 1*(2), 55–68. [Online] Available: www.cjsm.com.

Meenaghan, T. (1994). Point of view: Ambush marketing—immoral or imaginative practice? *Journal of Advertising Research, 34*(5), 77–88.

Melchert, A. (1997, March). *8th World Swimming Championships, Perth, Australia, 8th–18th, January 1998 management plan*. Unpublished manuscript.

Mill, R. C. (1990). *Tourism: The international business*. Englewood Cliffs, NJ: Prentice Hall.

Mill, R. C., & Morrison, A. (1992). *The tourism system*. Englewood Cliffs, NJ: Prentice Hall.

Miller Brewing Company. (1992). *Good times: A guide to responsible event planning*. Milwaukee, WI: The Miller Brewing Company.

Mitchell, T. (1995). Worlds apart: An Egyptian village and the international tourism industry. *Middle East Report, 25*, 8–11.

Morgan, D. (1984). *Managing urban America*. Belmont, CA: Brooks/Cole Publishing Company.

Mount, J., & Leroux, C. (1994). Assessing the effects of a mega-event: A retrospective study of the impact of the Olympic Games on the Calgary business sector. *Festival Management & Event Tourism, 2*, 15–23.

Mount, J., & Niro, B. (1995). Sponsorship: An empirical study of its application to local business in a small town setting. *Festival Management and Event Tourism, 2*(3/4), 167–175.

Mullen, L. (1998). Houston's NFL odds seen rising. *Street and Smith's Sports Business Journal*, September 21–27, 1(22), p. 3.

Mullin, B., Hardy, S., & Sutton, W. (2000). *Sport marketing*. Champaign, IL: Human Kinetics Publishers.

National Society for Park Resources (1998, Spring/Summer). The different faces of tourism [National Society for Park Resources Newsletter]. Ashburn, VA: National Recreation and Park Association.

Nelson, R. R. (October 1996). *The rising costs associated with attracting and retaining professional sports franchises*. Paper presented at the Sport in the City International Symposium, University of Memphis. Memphis, TN.

Newman, R. (1989). The convention and visitors bureau: An important resource in local Marketing. *Travel and Tourism Executive Report, 9*(1,2), 3.

Ocean Action Durban. Available online: www.oceanaction.co.za/html/body_dur_schedule.htm [1998, September 9].

Oldenburg, A. (1999). Spending a fortune for fun. USA Today, April 2, E1–E2.

Oneal, M., Finch, P., Hamilton, J. O., & Hammonds, K. (1987, August). Nothing sells like sports. *Business Week*, 48–53.

Osterland, A. (1995, February 14). Field of nightmares. *Financial World*, 105–107.

Parkhouse, B. (Ed.). (1996). *The management of sport: Its foundation and application*. St. Louis, MO: Mosby-Year Book, Inc.

Pearce, P. (1988). *The Ulysses factor: Evaluating visitors in tourist settings*. New York, NY: Springer Verlag.

Peterson, K., & Crayton, C. (1995). The effect of an economic impact study on sponsorship development of a festival. *Festival Management and Event Tourism, 2*(3/4), 185–190.

Phares, D. (1996*). Sports under the arch: St. Louis teams, venues and public funds*. Unpublished manuscript, University of Missouri-St. Louis.

Pickard, T. (1999). Sport industry shows potential for boosting area economically. *Syracuse Herald American*, Sunday March 14, p. D3.

Piirto Heath, R. (1997). You can buy a thrill: Chasing the ultimate rush. American Demographics, June, www.demographics.com/publications/ad/97_ad/9706_ad/ad970631.htm

Pike Masteralexis, L., Barr, C. A., & Hums, M. A. (1998). *Principles and practices of sport management*. Gaithersburg, MD: Aspen Publishing, Inc.

Pitts, B. G., Fielding, L. W., & Miller, L. K. (1994). Industry segmentation theory and the sport industry: Developing a sport industry segment model. *Sport Marketing Quarterly, 3*(1),15–24.

Plog, S. (March 1972). *Why destination areas rise and fall in popularity*. Paper presented to the Southern California chapter of The Travel and Tourism Research Association, San Diego.

Population Council (1999). Population momentum. www.popcouncil.org/pop_momentum.html

Population Information Network (1994). World population growth from year 0 to stabilization. Gopher://gopher.undp.org/00/ungophers/popin/wdtrends/histor__Gopher://gopher.undp.org/00/ungophers/popin/wdtrends/histor_

Riley, R. (1995). Prestige worthy tourist behavior. *Annals of Tourism Research, 22*, 3, 630–649.

Richardson, S., Long, P. & Perdue, R. (1989). The Importance of Economic Impact to Municipal Recreation Programming, *Journal of Park and Recreation Administration*, 6(4), pp. 65–78.

Rickman, D. & Schwer, R. K. (1995). A comparison of the multipliers of IMPLAN, REMI, and RIMS II: Benchmarking ready-made models for comparison. *The Annals of Regional Sciences*, 29, 363–74.

Ritchie, J. R. B., & Aitken, C. E. (1984). Assessing the impacts of the 1988 Olympic Winter Games: The research problem and initial results. *Journal of Travel Research, 22*(2), 17–25.

Ritchie, J. R. B., & Smith, B. H. (1991). The impact of a mega-event on host region awareness: A longitudinal study. *Journal of Travel Research, 30*(1), 3–10.

Robinson, J. (1998). Take me out to the opera. www.demographics.com/publications/ad/98_ad/9810_ad/ad981010.htm

Roche, M. (1991). *Mega-events and urban policy: A study of Sheffield's World Student Games 1991*. Unpublished manuscript, Policy Studies Center, University of Sheffield, Sheffield.

Roche, M. (1994). Mega-events and urban policy. Annals of Tourism Research, Vol. 21, pp. 1–19.

Rosentraub, M., Swindell, D., Przybylski, D., & Mullins, D. (1994). Sport and downtown development strategy: If you build it, will jobs come? *Journal of Urban Affairs*, 16, 221–239.

Sadker, M., Sadker, D. (1994). *Failing at Fairness : How Our Schools Cheat Girls*. New York, Simon and Scheuster, Inc.

Sandler, D. M. and Shani, D. (1989) "Olympic Sponsorship vs 'Ambush' Marketing: Who Gets the Gold?" *Journal of Advertising Research*, Vol. 11 Aug/Sep, pp. 9–14.

Schaffir, W (1988). Introduction. In *Getting value from strategic planning* [Research Report No. 915]. New York: The Conference Board. p. 96–104.

Schmader, S. W., & Jackson, R. (1997). *Special events: inside and out.* Champaign, IL: Sagamore Publishing.

Schor, J. (1991). The overworked American: The unexpected decline in leisure. Basic Books, New York, NY.

Seagle, E., Smith, R., & Dalton, L. (1992). *Internships in recreation and leisure services: A practical guide for students.* State College, PA: Venture Publishing.

Seaton, A. V., & Bennett, M.M. (1998). *Marketing tourism products.* London: International Thomson Business Press.

Shelton, C. (1991). Funding strategies for women's sports. *The Journal of Physical Education, Recreation and Dance, 62*(3), 51–54.

Skirstad, B. (1996). Place and function of the sports club. Proceedings *of the 4th European Congress on Sport Management.* European Society for Sport Management, Montpellier, France. p. 38–43.

Smith, S. H. & McLean, D. D., (1988). *ABC's of Grantsmanship.* Reston: VA. American Association for Leisure and Recreation.

Space future: Tourism or taxes [Online]. (1998). Available: www.spacefuture.com/tourism/taxes.shtml.

Pitzer, A. *Sports Illustrated,* (1995). Volume 83, (4), pp. 18–24.

Starr, N (1993). *Viewpoint: An introduction to travel, tourism, and hospitality.* Boston: Houghton Mifflin.

Stotlar, D. K., & Kadlecek, J. C. (1993, April). What's in it for me? *Athletic Business, 29,* 32–36.

Sutton, W., McDonald, M., & Milne, G. (1997). Creating and fostering fan identification in professional sports. *Sport Marketing Quarterly, 5*(1), 23–34.

Taylor, P. (1989). *Final report: Inquiry into the Hillsborough Stadium disaster.* City of Sheffield, England.

Ten Kate, N. (1995). No pain, no gain. American Demographics (November) www.demographics.com/publications/ad/95_ad/9511_ad/ad824.htm

Terrazas, M. (1995). Let the games begin. *American City and County, 110* (10), 24–28.

Texas Department of Economic Development (1997). Tourism development tip sheet: Sports tourism [Online]. Available at: www.ccta.org/travel/sportour 97.htm.

The World Cup soccer games finally come to America (1993, May 17). *Business America, 114* (10), 2–6.

Tom's Tourism Homepage (1998) WTO Statistical update. The biggest spenders. hubcap.clemson.edu/~prtm/wtoupdate.html

Tow, S. (1994). The benefits of sport-tourism. *Journal of Sport Tourism, 2*(1), 11–17.

Travel Industry Association of America (1998). Tourism Works for America—Report of TIA of America. www.tia.org/pubs/twfar98.stm

Travel Industry Association of America (1999). New Travel and Technology Report, www.tia.org.press/010899tech.stm).

Travel Industry Association of America. Fast facts: World tourism. www.tia.org/press/fastfacts6.htm.

Travel Weekly (June 6, 1998). p. 37

Travel Weekly (August 27, 1997). p. 13

Travel Weekly (October 9, 1997). p. 21

Turco, D. M., Riley, R.W., & Lee, S. H. (1999). Rolling down the river: The face of poor gamblers. Proceedings of Win, Lose or Draw: An International Symposium on Gambling, April 4–8, 1999, Omaha, NE.

Turco, D. M. (1995). Government as sponsor: State and local tax impacts generated by an international festival. *Festival Management & Event Tourism, 2*(3), 191–195.

Turco, D. M. (1994). *Residents' attitudes aoward the 1993 Kodak Albuquerque International Balloon Fiesta* [Technical report prepared for the AIBF, Inc.]. Albuquerque, NM.

Turco, D. M. (1994, December). Event sponsorship: Effects on consumer brand loyalty and consumption. *Sport Marketing Quarterly*, 42–45.

Turco, D. M. (1997). Measuring the economic and fiscal impacts of state high school sport championships. *Sport Marketing Quarterly, 6*(3), 49–53.

Turco, D. M. (1999). The state of tobacco sponsorship in sport. *Sport Marketing Quarterly, 8*(1), 35–38.

Turco, D. M. & Bretting, J. G. (1991, October). Financing urban park and recreation services: A look towards the 1990's. *Journal of Physical Education and Recreation* , 23.

Turco, D. M., & Eisenhardt, H. (1998). Exploring the sport-tourism connection. *ICHPER.SD Journal, 34*(2), 25–27.

Turco, D. M. & Kelsey, C. W. (1992). *Measuring the economic impact of special events*. Arlington, VA: NRPA.

Turco, D. M. & Ostrosky, T. (1997). Touchdowns and fumbles: Urban investments in NFL franchises. *Cyber-Journal of Sport Marketing, 1*(3), 100–110. Available online: www.cjsm.com.

U.S. Census Bureau (1999). World population profile: 1998 highlights.

United Nations Population Division (Unknown). Population prospects as assessed in 1994. New York: United Nations

Vogel, H., 1992, Travel and lodging industry marketing seminar: Managing marketing and sales automation for profit, *World Travel Market*, 17–18 November, Crafton Hotel, London.

Verner, B. (1996). Experiential learning through field experiences: Internships and practica. In B. Parkhouse (Ed.), *The management of sport: its foundation and application*. St. Louis, MO: Mosby-Year Book, Inc.

Wardell, D. The unknown online travel client, Travel Weekly, Feb. 26, p. 30.

Watt, D. C. (1992). *Leisure and tourism events management and organization manual*. Essex, UK: Longman Information and Reference.

Welcome to the 1998 Castle Lite Two Oceans Marathon!! [Online]. Available: www.twooceansmarathon.org.za/intro.htm [1998, March 3].

Weppler, K. A., & McCarville, R. E. (1994). *Understanding organizational buying behavior to secure sponsorship*. Unpublished undergraduate thesis, University of Waterloo, Waterloo, ON.

Weppler, K. A., & McCarville, R. E. (1995). Understanding organizational buying behavior to secure sponsorship. *Festival Management and Event Tourism, 2*(3/4), 139–148.

Whitson, D., & Macintosh, D. (1993). Becoming a world-class city: Hallmark events and sport franchises in the growth strategies of western Canadian cities. Sociology

Wholistic Consulting and Development in collaboration with the Department of Geography and Environmental Studies, University of Durban Westville (2000). Socio Economic Impact Study of the Vodacom Beach Africa Festival 2000, Unpublished Report).

Wicks, B. E., and Fesenmaier, D. R. (1995). Assessment of market potential for special events: A midwestern case study. Festival Management and Event Tourism, 3(1): 25–31.

Wilkinson, D. G. (1988). *A guide to effective event management and marketing*. Willowdale, Ontario: The Event Management and Marketing Institute.

Williams, P., & Harris, L. (1988). A framework for marketing ethnocultural communities and festivals. Unpublished report to the Secretary of State Multiculturalism, Ottawa.

World Tourism Organization (1997). 2020 vision predicts tourism as antidote to technology. www.world-tourism.org/newslett/nov97/vis2020.htm.

World Tourism Organization (1997). Travel to surge in the 21st century.

World Tourism Organization (1998). Hot tourism trends for 21st century.

World Tourism Organization (1998). Snow tourism threatened by global warming www.world-tourism.org/newslett/mayjun98/snowtou.htm __www.world-tourism.org/newslett/mayjun98/snowtou.htm_

World Tourism Organization (1999) What we offer? www.world-tourism.org/Offer.htm www.world-tourism.org/Offer.htm_

World Tourism Organization (1999). Results prove strength of tourism.

World Tourism Organization Business Council (1998). Leisure time squeeze will hot tourism. www.world-tourism.org/pressrel/1611–981.htm)

World Tourism Organization. (1991, June 28). Draft of the International Conference on Travel and Tourism Statistics: Ottawa Conference Resolutions. Available at www.worldtourism.org.

Wright, J. 1998. "EZ Links golf, Inc. offers instant tee times on the Internet" www.hospitalitynet.nl.news/article/11313566.htm

www.census.gov/ipc/www/wp98001.html

www.muc.edu/pe/gsmn197.htm

www.world- __www.world-_tourism.org/newslett/febmar99/1998res.htm

www.world- __www.world-_tourism.org/newslett/julaug98/OCEANS.htm.

www.world-tourism.org/newslett/nov97/travel.htm.

Yamane, T. (1967). *Elementary sampling theory*. Englewood Cliffs, NJ: Prentice-Hall.

Zeithaml, V. A., Parasuraman, A., & Berry, L. L. (1990). *Delivering quality service: balancing customer perceptions and expectations*. New York: The Free Press.

Zipp, J. (1996). The economic impact of the baseball strike of 1994. *Urban Affairs Review* 32(2), Nov., p. 157.

Index

A

Advertising Age, 95

Amateur Athletic Union (AAU), 57

Americans with Disabilities Act, 49, 132–133

Anheuser-Bush, 167, 174

Annals of Tourism Research, 94

Antarctica, 238

Arnold, M., 195–196, 201

ASA Men's Fast Pitch Softball World Championship Tournament, 155

Asian Games (13ᵗʰ Annual), 151, 157

B

Baade, R. A., 217, 218

Baltimore Colts, 214

Barr, C. A., 118

baseball, 58–59

Baseball Hall of Fame. *See* Major League Baseball Hall of Fame

Berlonghi, A., 129

Berry, L. L., 86–87, 124

biking. *See* cycling

Bread Not Circuses, 75

C

Canada, 230, 231

Canadian Sport Tourism Initiative, 252

Cape Town (South Africa)

   events hosted by, 81

   sport tour in, 49

casinos, 219

Catherwood, D. W., 82, 84–85, 128, 143

Chicago Bulls, 6–7

Chicago Cubs, 247

Chicago White Sox, 215

China, 39, 230–231

Citrine, K., 130

Civil Rights Act (1972), Title IX, 49, 236

Cleveland Browns, 215

Coakley, J., 14–16

Cobb, S., 67

Coca-Cola Corporation, 167, 177

convention and visitor bureaus (CVBs), 38

Copeland, R. P., 168–169

Crompton, J. L., 45, 66, 92, 158

    on escapism, 45–46

cruises, 5, 32–33

Cuba, 39, 41

Cunningham, M. H., 148

cycling, 228

D

Delpy, L., 115, 232, 237, 248

Des Moines Golf and Country Club, 58

Detroit Lions, 216

Dominican Republic, 235

E

Earnhardt, Dale, 174

East Germany, 39

Elaboration Likelihood Model of Persuasion, 148

environmental impact assessment (EIA), 80

ESPN Extreme Games (X-Games), 27, 222, 238, 251

Expedia, 29

F

Farr, J., 183

Fesenmaier, D. R., 159

"Field of Dreams" baseball diamond, 6, 50

Fielding, L. W., 23

Fleck, L., 132

football (soccer) hooliganism, 123

G

gambling. *See* casinos; sport tourism, issues in, gambling

"Gatekeepers," 172–173

Gazel, R. C., 66

Germany, 235

Getz, D., 9–10, 76, 78–79, 80, 85, 99–100, 101, 104, 106, 110, 112, 114, 115, 116, 126, 129, 130, 140–142, 247
    on advertising, 135
    on business plans, 94–95
    on cash-flow management strategies, 119
    definition of public relations, 134
    on evaluating service quality, 124–125
    on evaluation, 144
    on event packaging goals, 137–138
    on goals of cost-revenue management, 117–118
    on portfolio-building process, 108–109
    on price structures, 126–127
    on volunteer selection process, 113
Gibson, H., 1
Goldblatt, J. J., 74, 115
golf, 222, 247
    cruises, 5
    tourism, 6
    and women, 236
Graham, S., 115, 131, 133, 137, 142
    "exclusivity plan," 129–131
Gran Prix Racing, 225
Green Bay, sport tour of, 52
Green Bay Packers, 51, 52, 55, 71
Green Bay Packers Hall of Fame, 52
Grube, J., 177
Gunn, C., 24

H
Hall, C. M., 124
Hawkins, D. E., 187–188
Hillsborough disaster, 123
Hong Kong, 231
Houston Oilers, 215
Hudman, L. E., 187–188
Hums, M. A., 118
Hungary, 231

I
IEG Sponsorship Report, 95
Illinois Department of Natural Resources, 180
Illinois Department of Transportation, 180
Illinois High School Association (IHSA), 56

India, 235

Indianapolis 500 Motor Speedway, 51

Indonesia, 231

International Conference on Travel and Tourism Statistics, 17

International Events Group, 167

International Olympic Committee (IOC), 82, 84
    Evaluation Commission, 83

International Tug of War, 58

Iraq, 39

Irwin, R. L., 169

ITN, 29

J

Jackson, R., 76, 77–78, 80, 81, 107

Japan, 235

Journal of Sport Tourism, 94, 204

Journal of Travel Research, 94

K

Kadlecek, J. C., 169–170

Kanz, Mike, 52

Kimberly-Clark Corporation, 170

Kodak Albuquerque International Balloon Fiesta, 150, 155, 158, 170,
    171, 175, 222
    sport tour, 160

Kodak Corporation, 177

Korean National Tourist Office, 231, 250

Kraus, R., 178

Kurtzman, J., 7

Kuzma, J. R., 169

L

Lamb, C. W., 92

League of Their Own, A, 51

Lee, S. H., 218–219

Leroux, C., 157–158

Letscher, M., 226, 228

Levine, J., 119
    on risk management, 122–123

Little Illini Orange & Blue Soccer Tournament, 72

Little League World Series, 70–71

Los Angeles Dodgers, 253

Los Angeles Rams, 216

Ludden, L., 183

M

Madden, P., 177

Major League Baseball Hall of Fame, 51, 247

Manchester United soccer team, 253

Mangin, P., 183

Manual for Cities Bidding for the Olympic Games, 82–83

Mayfield, T. L., 158

McCally, J. F., 169

McCarville, R. E., 166, 169, 172, 174

McCook, K., 169, 173–174

McDonald's Corporation, 177

Mexico, 230

Miami Dolphins, 215

Mill, R. C., 24

Miller, L. K., 23

Mitchell, Arthur, 90

Monday Night Football, 239

Morrison, A., 24

Mount, J., 157–158

Murdoch, Rupert, 253

N

NASCAR, 174, 177
   rise of the fan base, 248–250

National Association for Sport and Physical Education (NASPE), 187

National Basketball Association (NBA), 15, 217

National Bicycling Championships, 63–64

National Collegiate Athletic Association (NCAA), 81, 170, 217, 218, 249

National Football League (NFL), 214, 218
   revenue-sharing system, 214

National Olympic Committees (NOCs), 82

National Trampoline and Tumbling Games, 70

Nepal, 238

New Zealand
   "All Blacks" rugby team, 51
   sport tour in, 51
   and turmoil in sport tourism, 40

Newcastle United soccer team, 253

North American Convention and Tourism Bureaus, 250

North American Society for Sport Management (NASSM), 187

Norwegian Cruise Lines, 32–33
   themed cruises, 32–33

NTL Cable, 253

O

Oakland Raiders, 214

Olympics (Summer and Winter), 3, 14, 49, 53, 61, 75, 79, 122, 217, 225, 239, 249. *See also* Paralympic Games
    bid process for, 83–84
        bidding recommendations, 84–85
        event lobbying, 84
        formal presentations, 84
    in Calgary, 157–158
    Cape Town bid for, 74, 75
    and displacement of Atlanta residents, 222
    in Los Angeles, 127
    Senior, 51, 70
    Special, 70

Ostrosky, T., 214

P

Paci, Enzo, 241–242

Paralympic Games, 49, 70

Parasuraman, A., 86–87, 124

Parkhouse, B., 185

Pepsi Corporation, 167

Pike Masteralexis, L., 118, 123–124, 137

Pitts, B. G., 23

Plog, S., 48

Poland, 231

Pontiac Silverdome, 216

price fixing, 166

PRIZM, 91

professional preparation in sport tourism, 183–184
    academic programs, 184–185
    core content of undergraduate programs, 186–188
    and Graduate Record Examination (GRE) scores, 195–196
    graduate school, 193–196
    and networking, 201
        evaluating, 202–204
        preconference, 201–202
    and professional associations, 200–201
    professional organizations, 204–212
    and seeking employment, 196–199
    service learning, 188–192
    websites
        for internships and jobs, 192–193
        for sports management/tourism programs, 185–186

program evaluation and review techniques (PERT), 103–104
Public Health Smoking Act (1970), 177

R
Request for Proposals (RFPs), 82
resorts, 5–6
return on investment (ROI), 56, 216, 217
Reynolds Tobacco Company, 176–177
Rickman, D., 66
Riley, R., 173–174
Riley, R. W., 218–219
Ritchie, J. R. B., 157, 158
Riverfront Stadium, 216
Robert Trent Jones Golf Trail, 5
Robinson, J., 249

S
Sadker, D., 196
Sadker, M., 196
St. Louis Cardinals, 216
St. Louis Rams, 216, 217
Schaffir, W., 100
Schmader, S. W., 76, 77–78, 80, 81, 107
Schwer, R. K., 66
Shanklin, W. L., 169
Singapore, 231
skiing, 247–248
Smith, B. H., 157, 158
South Africa, 51, 82, 231. *See also* Cape Town
Southern Cross University, 186
sport
    definitions, 16
    economic costs in, 58–59
    institutionalized, 15
    multiple dimensions of, 14–17
    and technology, 228
sport tourism. *See also* professional preparation in sport tourism; sport tourism, economic impact of; sport tourism, evaluation of; sport tourism events; sport tourism events, strategies for implementation; sport tourism, financing of; sport tourism, future directions; sport tourism industry; sport tourism, issues in; sport tourism services, problems of; sport tourism system
    annual growth rate, 2

   definition, 1–3
      hard, 8
      model, 7–8
      soft, 8–9
   as distinct market niche, 48–49
      and sport access to society, 49
      and sport prominence in society, 49–51
   economic power of, 250
   expenditures on, 2
   intensity of involvement in, 10–14
   marketplace, 250–253
   models, 4–7. *See also* sport-event tourism model
      Getty, 9
   primary attractions, 36
      human-contrived, 37
      human-reproduced, 37
      natural resource-based, 36
   relationships, 3–4
   secondary attractions, 37–38
      destination promotions, 38
      information services, 38–39
   supplier, 12–14
sport tourism, economic impact of, 53–54
   benefits of, 55–56
   and community development, 57–58
   and consumer market profile, 57
   econometric models, 65–66
      criticisms of, 66
      input-output (IO), 65–66
   enhancing an organization's image, 57
   importance of research on, 56–57
   indirect, 54
   issues in impact research, 66–67
      multipliers, 67–69
      spending patterns, 70–71
   spatial distribution of spending, 54–55
   steps in conducting impact research, 59
      Step 1. Determine scope of study, 59–60
      Step 2. Select data collection strategy, 61–63
      Step 3. Compute direct economic impact, 63–64
sport tourism, evaluation of, 147, 161
   determination of sport tourist groups, 156
   issues in, 150–151

overview of field survey approaches, 151–153

and longitudinal research approaches, 157–158

and promotional effectiveness research, 159

and residents' perceptions of sport tourism, 158–159

and sampling, 153–155

    sample size, 154

sponsorship evaluation, 148–150

and sport tourist satisfaction, 148

survey location, 155

sport tourism events, 73, 109–110. *See also* sport tourism events, strategies for implementation

bidding considerations, 81–82

    bid book requirements, 82–83

    process, 82

definition, 74

factors related to poor events, 107

    incompetent personnel, 107

    indifferent marketing, 107

    inferior physical environment, 108

    insufficient creativity, 107

    insufficient funding, 108

    poor timing, 108

    too much, too often, 108

feasibility study, 76

    questions considered in, 76–80

    "Yes" study, 81

formal appraisal of need to host an event, 75–76

future considerations, 108–109

importance of research, 74

informal assessment if need to host event, 74–75

location considerations, 104

    location, 105–107

    setting, 105

and market segments, 88–90

organizational structure, 101–102

    project management team, 103

    timeline considerations, 103–104

planning considerations, 85

    market, 86–88

    strategic planning considerations, 95. *See also* SWOT, analysis; SWOT, situational analysis

    identifying aims and objectives, 96

    identifying mission statement, 95

sport tourism events, strategies for implementation, 111. *See also* volunteer
    services subcommittee for the 8th World Swimming Championships
   administrative strategies, 112, 144–145
     personnel and volunteers, 112–116
   budget types, 118
   community involvement strategies, 124
   cost-revenue management, 117–118
   event evaluation strategies, 143–144
   financial strategies, 116–117
   legal considerations, 119–122
   operations plan, 125
     accommodations, 132–134
     accreditation, 132
     advertising, 135–137
     alcohol policy, 129
     communications, 126
     concessions and food services, 131
     facilities, 127–128
     medical services, 125–126
     public relations (marketing) operations, 134–138
     sanitation/refuse operations, 131–132
     security/emergency procedures, 128–129
     special needs accommodations, 132–133
     ticket, 126–127
     transportation and parking, 129–131
   quality service strategies, 124–125
     training for, 125
   risk management, 122
     comprehensive, 122–124
     definition, 122
   sponsorship strategies, 139
     benefits of, 139
     importance of research, 139–140
     signage, logos, and graphics, 142–143
     sponsorship platforms, 140–142
     sponsorship proposal, 142
sport tourism, financing of, 163, 182
  and capital development, 178–179
  earned income fees and charges, classifications of, 165
  grants, 181
    databases for, 181
  for nonprofit organizations (NPOs), 179–181
  pricing policies, 166

discount, 166
   leisure services, 166–167
resources, 182
revenue sources, 163–164
   compulsory, 164–165
sponsorship, 167–168
   benefits, 169–170
   considerations, 174–175
   decision-making, 168–69, 172–174
   issues, 175–176
   six steps in, 170–172
   tobacco, 176–177
sport tourism, future directions, 225–226, 253
  and demographics, 232–236
  extreme sports, 238–240
  general tourism trends, 228–232
  geographical/environmental, 240–241
  and marketing, 245–48, 250–253
  and motivations/lifestyles, 236–238
  and technology, 241–245
  trends versus fads, 226–228
sport tourism industry, 23–24
sport tourism, issues in, 213
  gambling, 218–19
    Atlantic City versus Las Vegas, 219–220
    dog and horse racing, 220
    future of, 220–221
  host-guest interactions, 222–223
  overcommercialization of sport, 221–222
  urban sport-facility development, 214–218
sport tourism services, problems of, 41
  heterogeneity of service offerings, 44
  inseparability of production and consumption, 42–43
  intangibility of services, 41–42
  perishability of services, 43–44
sport tourism system, 24
  and consumers, 25–26
  and governmental politics, 24–25, 253
  internet travel services, 29–30
  and politics, 39–41
  retail travel agencies, 28–29
  and tour wholesalers, 28
    escorted travel packages, 28

    hotel travel packages, 28

    transportation sector, 30–31

        airlines, 31–32

        coach, 33

        cruise lines, 32–33

        destination services, 34–36

        infrastructure travel support, 33–34

        rental cars, 33

sport tourist, 10–12, 148

    behavior and modifications, 44–45

    determining groups, 155

    personality types

        allocentric, 48

        midcentric, 48

        psychocentric, 48

    push and pull factors, 45–48

Sport Tourist Destination Area (STDA), 92–94, 99, 100

    strategies, 94

sport-event tourism model, 9–10

    demand side, 10–12

    supply side, 12–14

sports bars, 35–36

Sports Marketplace, 95

Sports Sponsors Fact Book, 95

Sports Tourism International Council (STIC), 186, 204

Stotlar, D. K., 169–170

Super Twelve Rugby, 243, 253

Sutton, W. A., 169

SWOT (Strengths, Weaknesses, Opportunities, and Threats), 94

    analysis, 97, 99

    situational analysis, 99–101

T

Taylor, Peter, 123

Taylor, S. F., 148

Thailand, 231

Tibet, 238

tour operators, 28

tourism, 17, 20

    definition, 17–19

    domestic, 19

    fluctuations in the market, 25

    international, 19

national, 19

tourism sports

    hard definition, 9

    soft definition, 9

tourist categorizations, 20–22

tours, 5. *See also individually listed sport tours*

track and field, 247

Travel Industry Association of America (TIAA), 2

travel intermediaries, 27–28

Travel and Tourism Research Association, 94

Travelocity, 29

Turco, D., 173–174, 214, 218–219

U

Union of Soviet Socialist Republics (USSR), 39, 231

United States, 39, 165, 230, 235, 241, 247

    and consumer spending, 239

United States Department of Agriculture (USDA), 65

United States Department of Commerce Travel and Tourism Division, 68

United States Department of Labor, 198

University of Luton, 186

V

Vail, Colorado, and recruitment of minority skiers, 247–248

Values Attitudes and Lifestyles (VALS), 90–91, 238

Van Kirk, R. L., 82, 84–85, 128, 143

Verner, B., 189

Vodacom Beach (Africa) sport tour, 98

volunteer services subcommittee for the 8th World Swimming Championships, 116

    duty statements, 116

W

Walt Disney Company/Walt Disney World, 6, 57, 71, 251, 253

Weinberg, D., 67

Weppler, K. A., 172, 174

WGN Broadcasting, 253

Wicks, B. E., 159

Wilkinson, D. G., 81, 112, 113, 117, 125, 126, 127, 131, 144

    on understanding the media, 134–135

World Cup, 217, 218, 225, 226, 239

World Cup Travel Services, 138

World Horseshoe Tournament, 58, 70

world population growth, 233–34

World Series of Little League baseball, 221

World Tourism Organization (WTO), 17, 19, 49, 226, 228–230, 237–238, 240

   Congress on Snow and Winter Sports Tourism (1998), 241

World Tourism Organization Business Council, 240

Z

Zauhar, J., 7

Zeithaml, V. A., 86–87, 124

zero-based budgeting (ZBB), 118

Zipp, J., 58–59

Zoreda, Jose Luis, 240

About the Authors

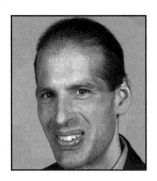

Douglas Michele Turco is professor of Kinnesiology and Recreation at Illinois State University. His primary research interests are in sport and tourism marketing, event economic impact assessment, and market research. He has made numerous national and international presentations and is the author or co-author of articles that appear in *Sport Marketing Quarterly, Journal of Tourism Studies, Journal of Travel Research, and Current Issues in Tourism*. He co-authored the book, *Sport and Event Marketing*, as well as several other books, book chapters, and conference proceedings. Dr. Turco earned his academic degrees from the University of Wisconsin-LaCrosse and the University of New Mexico.

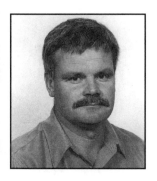

Roger Riley is an associate professor in the Department of Physical Education and Recreation at Winona State University in Minnesota. His research and writing encompasses a wide range of tourism related topics including sports tourism, movie-induced tourism, and "edge" tourism. In addition, he has a continuing interest in qualitative research methods. Dr. Riley was born and raised in New Zealand and held academic positions at Illinois State University and Ithaca College after receiving degrees from the University of Wisconsin-La Crosse and Texas A&M University.

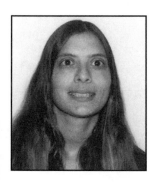

Kamilla Swart is currently account director for an international sport marketing company, Octagon South Africa, where she manages event tourism strategy. Swart has worked to develop South Africa's first post-secondary curricula devoted to sport tourism and has represented the Olympic Bid Company at the Paralympic Games and the World Athletic Championships. She is co-author of the first U.S. text on sport tourism, and her manuscripts have been published in the *Journal of Sport Tourism* and *Visions in Leisure and Business*. Dr. Swart earned a masters degree in Human Movement Studies from Rhodes University, South Africa and a doctoral degree in Curriculum and Instruction from Illinois State University.